WHEN VIOLENCE ERUPTS
A Survival Guide for Emergency Responders

▼ ▼

WHEN VIOLENCE ERUPTS
A Survival Guide for Emergency Responders

DENNIS R. KREBS
LIEUTENANT

Baltimore County Fire Department
Baltimore County, Maryland

KENNETH C. HENRY
DISTRICT CHIEF

Hillsborough County Fire Department
Hillsborough County, Florida

MARK B. GABRIELE
SERGEANT

Maryland State Police
Pikesville, Maryland

with 166 illustrations

THE C. V. MOSBY COMPANY
St. Louis ▼ Baltimore ▼ Philadelphia ▼ Toronto   1990

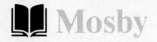

Editor: Richard A. Weimer
Assistant Editor: Adrianne H. Cochran
Project Manager: Carol Sullivan Wiseman
Production Editor: Linda McKinley
Book Designer: Susan E. Lane

Cover Photograph: Rick Brady

To the best of their ability, the authors have ensured that all events and facts are accurate. Some protocols may vary according to local standards. Mentions and photographs of equipment are not endorsements of the material.

The C.V. Mosby Company
11830 Westline Industrial Drive, St. Louis, Missouri 63146

Library of Congress Cataloging in Publication Data

Krebs, Dennis R.
    When violence erupts: a survival guide for emergency responders/
Dennis R. Krebs, Kenneth C. Henry, Mark B. Gabriele.
        p.   cm.
    Includes bibliographical references.
    ISBN 0-8016-6195-1
    1. Emergency medical personnel—Safety measures.   2. Emergency medical personnel—Crimes against—Prevention.   I. Henry, Kenneth C.   II. Gabriele, Mark B.   III. Title.
    RC86.7.K73   1990
    362.1'8—dc20   89-13769
                                                CIP

C/D/D   9   8   7   6   5   4   3

AUTHORS' NOTE

It is not the authors' intention to make you crawl up to every car, sneak up to every house, and not touch anything you didn't bring with you. Not everyone out there intends to hurt you. The majority of people sincerely appreciate your assistance—people will still send thank you cards to the station and tell their friends what a great job you did for them. There *are* a lot of nice people out there!

When you arrive on the scene of your next emergency, go about your business as usual. However, if something about the situation makes you feel uncomfortable, back off and think about it.

▼ ▼

FOREWORD

Over the many years I have been involved in emergency medical services, I have seen advances in technology, new training programs, and many publications that have had a positive impact on emergency response personnel and their practices. None of these has impressed me as having as significant an impact on personnel as the Medical Emergency Defense and Incident Control Seminar (MEDIC), which was developed and taught by Dennis Krebs and Mark Gabriele. The first time I saw the program, I knew the course materials had to be captured in print so that all emergency care personnel could benefit from the information.

That was in 1984. Over the following years the need for such a book has escalated. Violence in the home and on the street has become a significant hazard to emergency response personnel. This hazard not only exists in the urban setting, as one would imagine, but also has spread to suburbia and even the rural parts of our country.

Emergency response personnel are not attuned to worrying about their own safety. Their training concentrates on preparing them to help others. Most emergency response personnel are under the impression that they are viewed by their constituency as "helpers." This image gives them the false security that they are immune to harm from those they help. Unfortunately, this is not the case. In many situations, emergency response personnel encounter unexpectedly hostile environments or are innocent victims of a violent situation.

Obviously, there is a need to increase the awareness of our personnel so that they have a high index of suspicion when responding to incidents and know what to do when they encounter dangerous situations. Because of time constraints, current emergency medical services training programs do not include much of this training. That is why the MEDIC program has been so valuable to those who have had the opportunity to attend. Besides providing street-survival training, this book is valuable and an excellent resource because the authors "have been there." They have experienced the dangers of emergency response firsthand. Over the years of providing training with the MEDIC seminar, the authors have also gained more information from the experiences of their students, which they have incorporated into the program.

When the authors became involved in emergency services, they dedicated their lives to the saving of other lives. Like all emergency care providers, they felt that the lives they influenced would be those of their patients and their patients' families. Through the development of the MEDIC training seminar, and finally, with the writing of this textbook, they have expanded their role of saving lives to include those of their fellow responders. They will have an impact on a much greater number of lives than they ever anticipated when they started their careers.

While I hope that all emergency care providers and response personnel will have an opportunity to read this book and benefit from the information, I hope that instructors will incorporate the applicable parts into their training programs so that all emergency response providers learn from the beginning to protect themselves. This book will enhance the safe practice of emergency response personnel and, in turn, keep them active and available to provide their valuable services to their communities.

MARY BETH MICHOS
ASSISTANT CHIEF
Chief, Emergency Medical Services Division
Montgomery County Department of Fire and Rescue Services
Montgomery County, Maryland

PREFACE

While working a daylight tour of duty in early 1983, Dennis Krebs was assigned to the medic unit operating out of the Towson Fire Station in Baltimore County, Maryland. The majority of the unit's first-due response district was a white-collar business community surrounded by usually quiet, upper-middle class and affluent residential areas.

Shortly after Krebs assumed the duty, the dispatcher announced the first call for the tour: "Medic 1, respond to Charles Street and Kenilworth Drive for a possible heart attack; man reported slumped over the steering wheel." When the medic unit arrived on the scene, Krebs and his partner found the driver slumped over the steering wheel in his car, which was stopped on the shoulder of the road. As they approached the driver's side of the vehicle, there was a strong odor of alcohol. Feeling that it was "just another drunk," Krebs reached through the open window, touched the occupant on the shoulder, and told him to "Wake up."

He was nearly killed when the subject sat up with a .357 Magnum in his hand and attempted to shoot Krebs in the face. Fortunately a state trooper had approached the vehicle from the opposite side and was able to disarm the subject before anyone was harmed.

Could an incident similar to this happen to you? It may have already happened in your area. Some examples from around the nation include the following:

> ▶ Baltimore, Maryland: Fire department medical personnel knocked on the front door of a house and were greeted by two arrows shot through the closed door.[1]

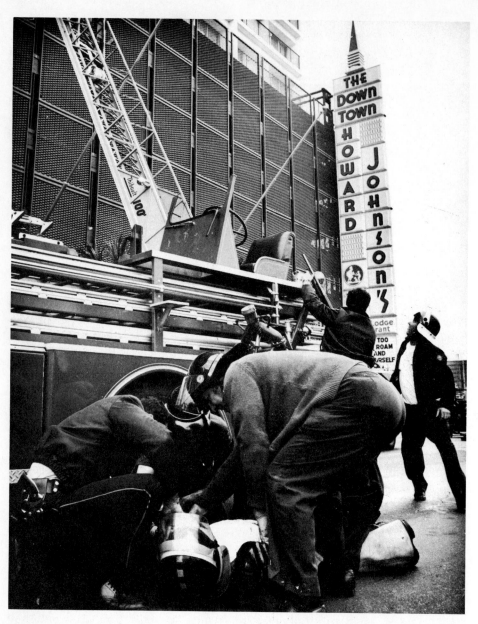

Firefighters and police officers under gunfire while attempting to extinguish multiple fires set by a sniper/arsonist at a hotel. Four emergency services personnel were killed and six were wounded.[3] (*Courtesy G.E. Arnold, The States-Item, Gretna, La.*)

▶ Bellevue, Tennessee: Responding to a request for assistance, a firefighter was attacked and kidnapped. The incident ended with a dead
  firefighter.[2]

▶ New Orleans, Louisiana: Firefighters and police officers were under
  gunfire while extinguishing multiple fires set by a sniper/arsonist at
  a Howard Johnson hotel. Four emergency services personnel were
  killed, and six were wounded.[3]

▶ Pittsburgh, Pennsylvania: Paramedics were attacked and injured
  while attempting to provide medical assistance to the victim of a
  domestic disturbance. The assailant had objected to their giving
  care.[4]

▶ San Ysidro, California: Engine crew members were pinned down by
  gunfire for 90 minutes during the McDonald's massacre.[5]

▶ Philadelphia, Pennsylvania: Five firefighters were wounded when
  they were caught in a cross-fire during a gun battle between police
  and the radical group MOVE.

Stories of similar near-fatal incidents to emergency service providers
are heard from personnel in agencies of every size and location. For example, 180 ambulance personnel were assaulted in Chicago during 1988.[6]
These incidents are increasing in frequency and can happen anywhere,
anytime, and within any socioeconomic group. Ghetto areas are no longer
the only place where violent incidents occur. Residential neighborhoods,
which are usually quiet, frequently produce tense moments for fire and rescue personnel. Weapons can find their way into any hand, and violence is
not always selective of its victims.

Defending yourself against violence is not part of your job. However,
you need to know how to avoid violence when possible and how to protect
yourself when it erupts.

The purpose of this book is not to make you afraid to answer an
alarm; it is to help you reach a middle ground where you can function effectively and safely.

The first chapter will help you to understand the physical threat that
you face each time you respond to an emergency. It will challenge you to be
a *proactive* and not a *reactive* emergency services provider.

Chapters 2 through 4 cover highway incidents. The potential danger
involved in these incidents is of primary concern to the law enforcement
community, but it is seldom recognized by responders from other emergency services agencies, such as fire, rescue, and EMS. Chapter 2 identifies
incidents that indicate a need for caution and describes unit positioning
and personal precautions that you should take before leaving your unit.
Chapter 3 describes how to approach a vehicle, and Chapter 4 tells you how
to flee from an armed encounter.

Chapters 5 through 8 deal with incidents inside a structure. Topics include how to approach and enter a residence safely, how to deal with a do-

mestic quarrel, and how to handle medical emergencies in places of public assembly.

Do you know the difference between cover and concealment? Not knowing could cause you to lose your life. Examples of each are depicted in Chapter 9.

The news media mentions hostage situations in our country and abroad every day. First responders may be called on to respond to a hostage situation without any preparation on what to expect. Chapter 10 explains how to react when you are called to a hostage scene and, more important, how to survive if you become a hostage.

Do you understand your responsibilities at a reported bomb threat? How can you avoid booby traps? Can a tube of toothpaste or a man's wallet be lethal weapons? Read Chapter 11 to find out the answers to these questions.

Chapter 12 gives details on recognizing a clandestine drug lab. Without understanding the hazards associated with operations in and around the illegal drug lab, you may be exposed to chemicals that will kill you on contact or slowly destroy your life.

How do you defend yourself when you are physically attacked? Chapter 13 demonstrates several self-defense tactics that may save your life.

A new field of specialization is available to paramedics and emergency medical services personnel in many parts of the country. The duties of a typical SWAT medic are described in Chapter 14.

As far as the authors are aware, this is the first text to provide fire, rescue, and EMS personnel with comprehensive tactics for their personal safety. Use of these tactics cannot guarantee your safety, but they will increase your chance of survival *when violence erupts.*

DENNIS R. KREBS
KENNETH C. HENRY
MARK B. GABRIELE

ACKNOWLEDGMENTS

As with any book of this type, no one person can be credited with all of the work. We recognize the impact on this project of each person taking the time to talk with us before, during, or after one of our seminars. Those individuals that have shared their personal experiences on the street and given suggestions on how to make "the job" safer for all of us are too numerous to mention. It is impossible to express adequately what we feel in our hearts for all those brothers and sisters in the service who are sincerely concerned about a safe work environment. Please accept our efforts with this book as our thanks for your commitment.

A personal thanks from each of us to Assistant Chief Mary Beth Michos of the Montgomery County Department of Fire and Rescue Services, Maryland, for recognizing the need for a text such as this. Without her original belief in our abilities and constant support throughout the development of the text, this book may never have been completed.

We thank the many law enforcement agencies assisting in this project. Some that deserve specific recognition are Ray McKinnon with the Drug Enforcement Administration and George McCoy, deputy fire marshal of the Oregon State Fire Marshal's Office, for help with clandestine drug labs; Cliff Lund and the Bureau of Alcohol, Tobacco, and Firearms for helping with bombs and booby traps; Dennis Hill and Arlene Jenkins of the Baltimore City Police Department's Public Information Division for photographs of the many weapons being used in our streets; and the Federal Bureau of Investigation for the information on hostage situations and terrorism.

News agencies from around the country graciously provided news articles and photographs of the major incidents mentioned throughout the book. The *Perry County Times*, the *Sentinel*, *The Philadelphia Inquirer*, the *New Orleans States-Item*, and the Union-Tribune Publishing Company were especially helpful.

The material on soft body armor would not have been possible without the assistance of Thomas E. Bachner, Jr., and Louis H. Miner of E.I. Du Pont De Nemours and Company.

The tireless assistance of Stephen K. Erwin of the Rapides Parish Sheriff's Department EMTAC Team and Michael J. Essex of the Miami Fire Department made the chapter on SWAT medics possible.

Tools and equipment used in many of the descriptive photographs were provided by Clemens Industries, Inc.

We thank the many fire and rescue services from around the nation that answered our requests for information. Without their willingness to share critiques of past local incidents, present policies, and innovative standard operating procedures, this book would lack validity.

Paramedic Becky Bryant of the Hillsborough County Emergency Medical Services, Florida, critically read the draft copies of the manuscript (many chapters more than once). We appreciate her professional comments and stimulating discussion throughout this project.

The tedious task of proofreading was ably completed by RMC Billy-Ace Baker, OAE, USN (retired), and NCCS David A. Bodin, USN (retired), wordsmiths from Pensacola, Florida.

Finally, thanks to our families for their patience and understanding during the countless hours spent working on this book. We are fortunate to have wives as supportive and tolerant as Terry Krebs and Colleen Henry. They are special!

CONTENTS

APPENDIXES

A
SOFT BODY ARMOR 191

B
CHEMICALS USED IN CLANDESTINE DRUG LABS 195

C
EMTAC BASIC TRAINING CURRICULUM 203

D
EMTAC EQUIPMENT 207

▼   ▼

ABBREVIATIONS

ALS	Advanced Life Support
BDU	Battle Dress Uniform
BLS	Basic Life Support
DOT	Department of Transportation
ECG	Electrocardiogram
ERG	*Emergency Response Guidebook*
EMS	Emergency Medical Service
EMT	Emergency Medical Technician
EMTAC	Emergency Medical Tactical Response
FBI	Federal Bureau of Investigation
IBM	International Business Machines
IV	Intravenous
JEMS	*Journal of Emergency Medical Services*
K.E.D.	Kendrix Extrication Device
MAST	Military Antishock Trousers
mEq	Milliequivalent
mg	Milligrams

ml	Milliliter
mm	Millimeter
m/s	Meters per second
NATO	North Atlantic Treaty Organization
NFPA	National Fire Protection Association
OD	Olive-Drab
OIC	Officer in Charge
psi	Pounds per square inch
SWAT	Special Weapons and Tactics
TFC	Trooper First Class
TNT	Trinitrotoluene
UN	United Nations
U.S.	United States
VHF	Very High Frequency
WNYF	*With New York Firefighters*

WHEN VIOLENCE ERUPTS
A Survival Guide for Emergency Responders

▼ **1** ▼

THE THREAT AND THE NEED

Some incidents do not reflect a true picture of on-scene conditions when dispatched. The caller may neglect to inform the dispatcher that the reason a person is having "difficulty in breathing" is because the victim was hit in the throat with a baseball bat. "Severe lacerations" may really mean multiple razor cuts, and the "attempted suicide" victim with a single gunshot wound in the back should be questioned.

You should never be complacent when responding to a call in a normally quiet neighborhood. These areas spawn domestic fights; child, drug, and alcohol abuse; and similar problems. Violence occurs as frequently there as in those sections of town noted for high crime. Rural areas are experiencing rapid growth as inner city populations relocate and bring their inner city problems and attitudes to previously quiet suburbs.

These types of incidents occur on a daily basis throughout our country. Each incident is a possible threat to the safety of emergency service providers who are untrained in personal protection tactics.

Fire, rescue, and emergency medical service departments throughout the country are addressing the problem of violence in the community in different ways. Unfortunately, many are ignoring the issue. Fire departments in Houston and the city of Los Angeles are providing paramedics with soft body armor for personal protection should they find themselves in a violent situation. In Branford, Connecticut, the local union purchased bulletproof vests for firefighters who respond to shooting or stabbing incidents.[1] Other agencies authorize wearing soft body armor on duty if individuals purchase it with their own funds.

1

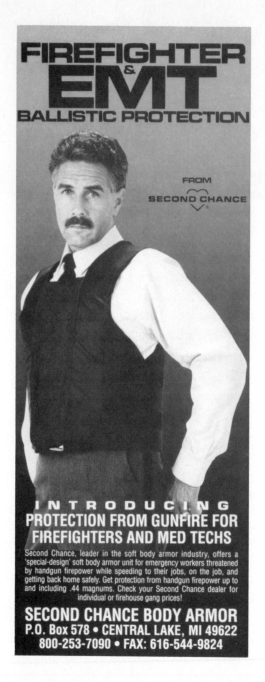

FIGURE 1-1

Brochure introducing ballistic protection for firefighters and emergency medical technicians that was distributed at the 1988 International Association of Fire Chiefs Conference. *(Courtesy Second Chance Body Armor, Inc., Central Lake, Mich.)*

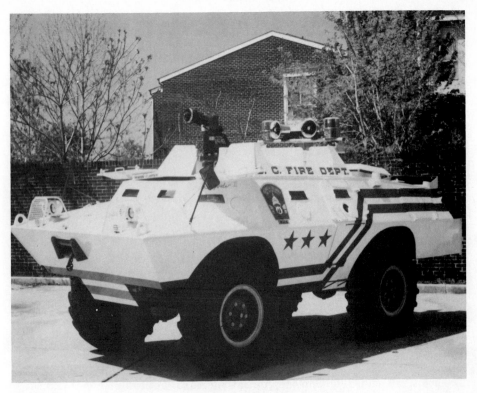

FIGURE 1-2
Armored personnel carrier operated by the District of Columbia Fire Department.

Progressive departments are providing fire, rescue, and emergency medical personnel with basic training classes, continuing education seminars, and hands-on training. They teach how to avoid violence and survive an incident that may suddenly escalate to the point where the situation can no longer be controlled.

Individual emergency service workers throughout the nation confidentially admit that they carry small-caliber handguns, blackjacks, knives, or other weapons for self-protection without department authorization.

Advertisements in professional periodicals are evidence that companies selling personal protection products recognize a potential market in fire, rescue, and emergency medical services (Figure 1-1).[2] Fabricators of armor-plated vehicles (Figure 1-2) are advertising antiterrorist cabs for fire apparatus in fire service trade publications.[3]

Emergency service personnel are constantly learning the hard way how to deal with situations that threaten their personal safety. Many of these experiences result in serious injury or death of the emergency service worker (Figure 1-3). This book provides the basic tactics for personal survival and will help you recognize those situations that could be fatal if

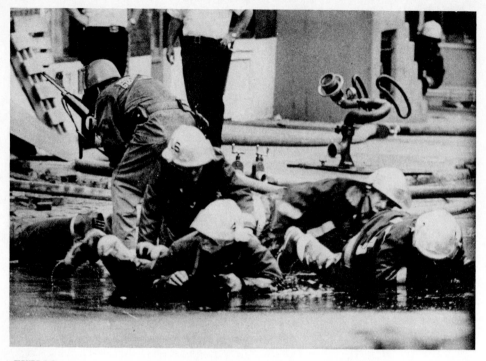

FIGURE 1-3
Firemen scramble for safety when gun battle breaks out between police and the radical group MOVE. *(Courtesy Wide World Photos, New York.)*

not handled properly. A routine call may suddenly turn into a violent situation and cause further injury to the patient, injury to the rescuer, or even death. If you practice the information presented in this book on a daily basis, you should survive the violence that may erupt when least expected.

The target audience is every emergency services responder who arrives on the scene before law enforcement personnel. To develop the necessary survival techniques, the responders need realistic survival training similar to the training received by law enforcement personnel. All emergency services agencies respond to potentially life-threatening situations daily; therefore, personnel from all responding agencies should receive the same training to protect themselves. Self-defense techniques are important for anyone faced with an aggressive patient. Force should be employed in some situations, and reasonable limits of force are necessary. These skills are not taught in most emergency medical technician or paramedic training programs.

Departments that encourage personnel to master survival techniques should experience a reduction in on-the-job injuries, long-term absences, and forced early retirements. A responder prepared to avoid or survive violence may experience less job-related stress and may be more receptive to assignment in a high-risk location.

The information in this text is not normally found in fire, rescue, or emergency medical services publications. This entire book is devoted to *your* survival. The information should not be shared with the general public. If the civilian community becomes aware of these survival tactics, the element of surprise will be lost and the tactics may be used against you.

Although this information will help many emergency services personnel avoid injury during the increasing number of violent incidents, the situation can still go awry. You can follow every safety precaution and still be injured or killed while answering an emergency. Many competent emergency services workers have died in the line of duty after doing everything right. Remember, if someone really wants to do you bodily harm, that person will find a way to accomplish the goal.

The threat is *there,* it is *real,* and it is *ever present.* The more the threat is understood, the better your chances of avoiding or surviving a violent situation.

I THOUGHT YOU WERE A COP!

Have you ever gone into a convenience store for coffee while on duty and received your coffee free because the clerk mistook your uniform for that of a police officer? How about the person from out of town who says, "Excuse me, officer, do you . . .?" This tourist also thought you were a police officer. No harm was done in either case; these were honest mistakes.

Many people mistake uniformed fire and rescue personnel for police officers. Compare the appearance of the people in Figure 1-4. Both persons have on blue pants, white shirts, name tags, and breast badges. Patches are visible on the sleeves. Both are holding flashlights and portable radios. Both have a bulge on their right hip; the police officer's is a gun, and the paramedic's is a pouch with scissors, forceps, and other instruments.

In fireground situations, firefighters are wearing protective clothing, which readily distinguishes them from police officers. As the first responders to a medical emergency, your protective clothing is usually in a side compartment of the medic unit or in the cab of the fire apparatus. Most departments consider it more professional to handle medical calls in clean uniform shirt and trousers rather than bunker gear.

The person whose consciousness has been altered by drugs or alcohol may confuse firefighters or medical personnel with law enforcement officers. This confusion caused by the similarity in uniforms could create a dangerous situation for the first responder.

For example, you arrive on the scene of a person slumped over the steering wheel. The medic unit has all warning lights operating, and the siren is still winding down as you get out of the unit. As you and your partner approach the vehicle, you are thinking, "I'm a paramedic. I'm here to help this person." You are unaware that this person was recently told by a judge that if he is caught driving while intoxicated again, "Bring your toothbrush, because you are going to be here awhile."

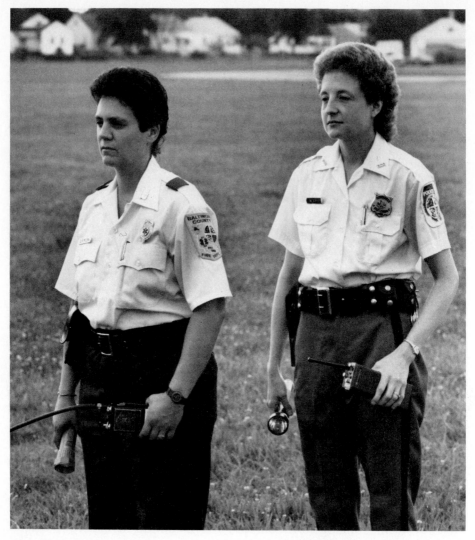

FIGURE 1-4
Uniformed fire and rescue personnel are easily mistaken for police officers.

The person sees flashing lights, the fact that they are red and white and not red and blue makes no difference. He heard a siren, saw the lights, and now he sees you standing there in uniform. He can't read the small print on the bottom of the patch that says **Paramedic** or **Fire Department**. Because of his recent trouble, all he sees is a police officer. You are thinking, "I'm here to help," and he is thinking, "Here is a cop." In his condition he expects to see a cop, and so he does. He knows the cop would not be there to *help* him.

In these situations the emergency services responder should anticipate receiving some form of aggressive action. The action may be verbal abuse or a physical attack, with or without the use of a weapon.

To prevent cases of mistaken identity, some departments have adopted the golf-style shirt as part of the uniform. These shirts do not have badges, patches, or collar devices. Only the department logo is printed on the left breast pocket. To soften their image, other departments authorize crew-neck pullover t-shirts with the department's initials over the left breast and on the back of the shirt.

I'M NOT A COP!

The nonchalant attitude of many firefighters, emergency medical technicians, and paramedics approaching an unknown situation places their personal safety in jeopardy. Their lives are constantly in danger as a result of their casual methods of approach. Someone may be waiting to provide the nonchalant responder with an attitude adjustment in the form of a gun in the face or a knife in the back.

When a call is dispatched for a shooting, stabbing, domestic assault, severe lacerations caused by a fight, or similar incident, law enforcement personnel are usually dispatched at the same time as the fire and rescue units. However, fire and rescue personnel frequently arrive on the scene before law enforcement personnel, especially in suburban and rural areas.

In rural areas a first alarm response from the fire or rescue services of two or three personnel may exceed the total number of law enforcement personnel patrolling the entire local jurisdiction. In urban areas, police assistance may not be available during peak trouble hours.

Until recently most personal survival training programs have been directed toward the law enforcement community. This causes a problem for fire, rescue, and emergency medical services personnel when they are forced into a dangerous situation while law enforcement personnel are en route to the scene.

THE ELEMENT OF SURPRISE

Most fire and rescue personnel do not have the authority to carry firearms, nor do they have the powers of arrest. The importance of maintaining an *element of surprise* must be recognized and practiced to offset this disadvantage. Many tactics and techniques not known by the general public are available to emergency services workers. The public will not expect you to take such actions. People will watch you approach a motor vehicle or a building and not know the systematic checks being analyzed in your mind. This element of surprise is the major form of self-protection available to fire and rescue personnel—its importance cannot be overemphasized.

CONTRARY TO PREVIOUS TRAINING

The key to every first responder, emergency medical technician, and paramedic training program has been, and in most cases still is, patient care. The fire and rescue services personnel fully realize the importance of rushing to the patient to stabilize the heart attack, handle the trauma, or treat the medical emergency. Stopping to think, "Hey, slow down, what about my safety?" is not considered macho.

Until recently this antiquated thinking permeated the entire fire service. Hazardous materials training has taught us that we can no longer rush right into the scene. Tactics courses now teach us to slow down. Check the nature of a vehicle's contents, write off the lost section of a structure, and don't compound the problem by committing personnel to body recovery until you know the cause of death.

Should a response to a hazardous situation receive the same cautious treatment as a response to a hazardous material? Yes! When responding to a gunshot wound, you may think MAST trousers,* IVs, and helicopter transport. You should be thinking, "Where is the person who pulled the trigger? Is the scene secure? Is the area safe to enter?" If you are shot on arrival, you are no help to the patient or to your partner.

A marked improvement in the caution used during responses to fire and hazardous materials emergencies has occurred over the past 5 years. Responses to medical emergencies should also change. Rushing right in is not always necessary. You should not charge through the door of a residence to aid a shooting or stabbing victim without law enforcement assistance. You should not remain in an area where verbal abuse could lead to physical abuse. Sometimes you will have the blood pressure cuff on a victim's arm and the stethoscope in your ears when the violence erupts. When this happens, you must leave the dangerous and violent situation that has developed. The victim you left behind may die—you will not.

When trouble occurs, you will not have time to put the victim on a backboard and strap him down in the proper manner. However, you may be able to grab the victim by the ankles and run. The victim may incur some additional injuries, but sometimes you have only two choices. Ask yourself, "Do I stay and continue to treat my patient while risking the possibility of being injured or killed, or do I leave the area immediately and, if time allows, drag the patient too?" Which is better for you? Our first concern is to look out for ourselves.

*Military Antishock Trousers.

▼   **SURVIVAL TIPS**   ▼

1 Even if you sincerely believe that your primary concern is for the patient and that these ideas are too radical, please do not stop reading.
2 This book will introduce you to ideas that can alter your attitude and help you stay alive to treat another patient on another day.
3 First responders in large cities are aware of increasing personal danger. Responders from suburbia may not expect sudden violence. Just because it has never happened to you does not mean it will not happen on your next call.
4 Unless your department has trained you to use a weapon and officially authorizes this practice, *do not* carry small-caliber handguns, blackjacks, knives, or other weapons for self-protection.
5 Possession of an unauthorized weapon may result in legal and civil liabilities for you. A weapon may give you a false sense of security and be used against you.
6 You must recognize the possibility of violence developing on every call.
7 NFPA 1500, *Fire Department Occupational Safety and Health Program,* requires your organization to provide you with training that will ensure your ability to perform your assigned duties safely.

2

HIGHWAY INCIDENTS AND YOUR APPROACH TO THE SCENE

Interstate highways were built to move goods and products necessary to maintain our standard of living, military personnel and equipment in time of a national emergency, and the motoring public. Regretfully, our highways are also used to transport illegal drugs, weapons, and other contraband, as well as criminals and illegal aliens.

The problems occurring on interstate highways may also be found on intrastate highways, city streets, narrow rural roads, and parking lots. Emergency responders must be aware of the potential danger on any call involving a motor vehicle, regardless of the location. The danger may range from minor physical abuse while attempting to treat an intoxicated driver to potential death if illegal drugs are discovered.

INCIDENTS THAT INDICATE A NEED FOR CAUTION

Traffic accidents, including those involving personal injury, usually are not dangerous situations for emergency services personnel who are responding to render assistance. However, many incidents should feel uncomfortable to you and indicate that caution should be exercised as you approach a stopped vehicle. These incidents may include the following:

▶ You arrive in a state-of-the-art emergency vehicle that has the loudest siren available. The maximum number of warning lights that the electrical system can support are operating. Heads are visible in the

11

vehicle, but no one turns around. There is no movement, only silence. This is not the normal response to your arrival. If someone in
the vehicle requires assistance and if someone in the vehicle is
awake and responsive, the normal reaction would be for the occupants to turn and look in your direction. The occupants should give
some indication of the problem and the location of anyone who requires assistance. If everyone in the vehicle continues to sit facing
forward without moving, your suspicions should be heightened.

▶ You arrive on the scene of a reported cardiac arrest that occurred in
a vehicle. You find the vehicle correctly parked on the side of the
right-of-way with no visible occupants. People seldom pull off to the
side of the road, put their vehicle in park, and lay down on the seat
and die. Because of the lack of time, the vehicle is usually found
stopped at an angle, against the guard rail, or in the ditch.

▶ You stop your unit to the rear of a vehicle reported to contain an injured person. Suddenly everyone gets out of the vehicle and starts
walking toward your unit. Could one of them be injured? Who called
for assistance?

▶ The driver of the vehicle adjusts the rearview or side mirror as you
exit the unit and watches your every move.

▶ The vehicle and the occupants appear out of place for the neighborhood. Could the crossing of invisible ethnic boundaries have caused
the existing situation? Could the situation escalate?

▶ Visible signs of violence such as guns, knives, or other weapons are
lying in the street. Where are the people who used them? Do they
have other weapons?

▶ You must enter a dimly lighted area or an area with limited exit (escape) routes. The area could be a deserted highway, a dark country
road, or an inner-city alley. Constantly maintain a sense of caution
when you are in precarious situations.

▶ You have a "gut feeling" that something is not right as you approach
the scene. Do not ignore this feeling. Analyze the cause before you
proceed.

As your level of concern increases, you should decide on a firm course of
action. Either continue the response and walk up to the vehicle as you normally would or call for law enforcement assistance and wait until the scene
is declared safe.

If you request law enforcement assistance each time you enter a questionable situation, you may soon develop a *crying wolf* reputation. This action is not conducive to a good relationship with the law enforcement community or a sign of professionalism. If emergency responders are trained to
carry out systematic approach procedures, it will not be necessary to call
for law enforcement assistance in most incidents. These procedures should
be used every time you experience the gut feeling that indicates the possibility of impending danger.

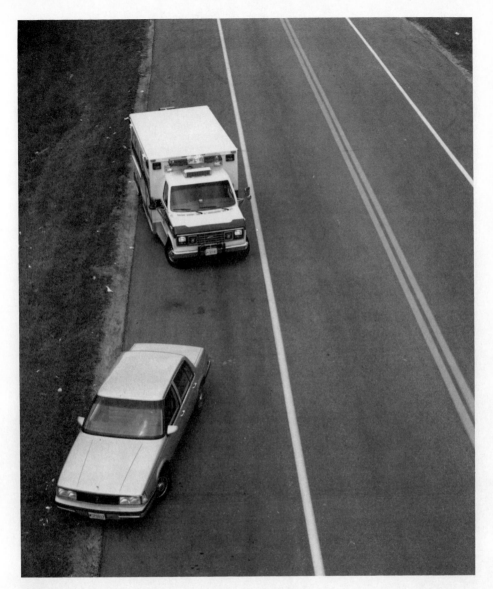

FIGURE 2-1
Position the unit a minimum of 15 feet to the rear of the stopped vehicle on a 10-degree angle to the left.

POSITIONING THE EMERGENCY RESPONSE UNIT

Whenever feasible, emergency service personnel should approach stopped vehicles from the rear. Exceptions to this rule will be discussed in Chapter 3. The unit should be positioned a minimum of 15 feet to the rear of the stopped vehicle on a 10-degree angle to the driver's side (Figure 2-1). As the unit stops, turn the wheels all the way to the left. In this position the

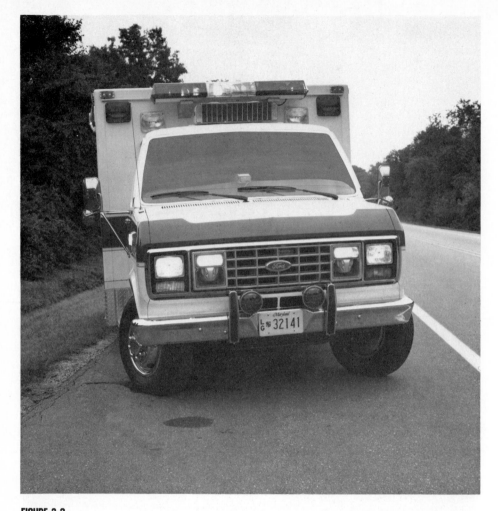

FIGURE 2-2
If gunfire erupts from the stopped vehicle before you pass the frontal plane of the
response unit, the turned wheels provide a protective area to hide behind.

engine block of most units and the wheels of all units can be used as protective areas should violence erupt.[1]

The density of the engine block and the wheels have the ability to stop
a bullet fired from a .357 Magnum, but a .22 caliber bullet may penetrate
the door area of the unit. If an occupant exits a stopped vehicle and begins
shooting at the emergency response team, the engine block and the wheel
areas offer the most protection to the responders (Figure 2-2).

Responders should always position the unit in a manner that will provide maximum protection. An improperly positioned unit can be a disadvantage to the responder who is required to approach a stopped vehicle, especially during a night approach.

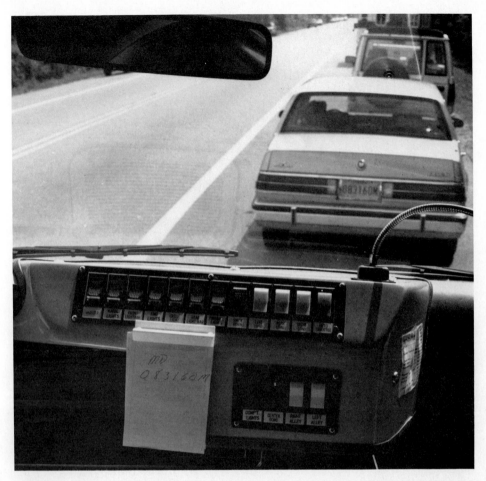

FIGURE 2-3
Before leaving the unit, write down the license number of the stopped vehicle and place the information in a predetermined location.

PERSONAL PREPARATIONS BEFORE LEAVING THE UNIT

When the unit arrives at the scene, do not leap out, grab the jump kit, and run up to the vehicle. Before leaving the unit, allow yourself several moments to inspect the scene for safety.

As the driver positions the unit, the person in the right front seat should be recording the license plate number of the stopped vehicle. Include the name of the state where the license tag was issued. If something happens to you and your partner, a written record of the vehicle exists. Before you leave the unit, place this information in a predetermined location, such as next to the radio (Figure 2-3). The advisability of giving this infor-

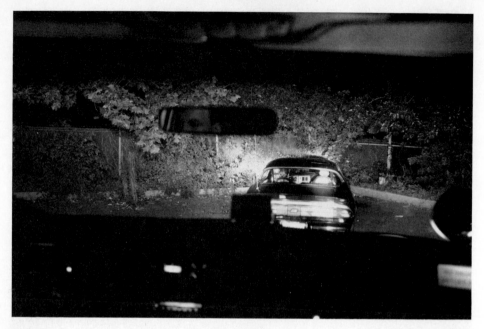

FIGURE 2-4
A normal medic unit light package will illuminate the interior and perimeter of the
vehicle.

mation to the communications dispatcher has been discussed with people
working in communications centers throughout the country. Their consen-
sus is that dispatchers may disregard the information as unimportant because they do not routinely receive this type of information. Writing the information down and placing it by the radio before leaving your unit is in
your own best interest.

When incidents occur after dark, the unit driver should use the high-
beam headlight setting to illuminate the interior and the perimeter of the
vehicle being approached. In units equipped with a spotlight, the driver
shines the light into the rearview mirror of the vehicle (Figure 2-4). This
will usually illuminate the interior of the passenger compartment. Emergency vehicles not equipped with spotlights may carry hand-held quartz
lights. As before, the driver aims the quartz light at the rearview mirror of
the vehicle. A properly aimed spotlight or quartz light will prevent the occupants from seeing the responder approach the rear of the vehicle.

When the emergency response unit is properly positioned, you can approach the driver's side of the vehicle without casting a shadow in the side
or rearview mirrors (Figure 2-5). Even though the unit lights are shining on
your back, the 10-degree angle of your unit to the vehicle casts your
shadow in the roadway instead of the vehicle's mirrors. Do not walk be-

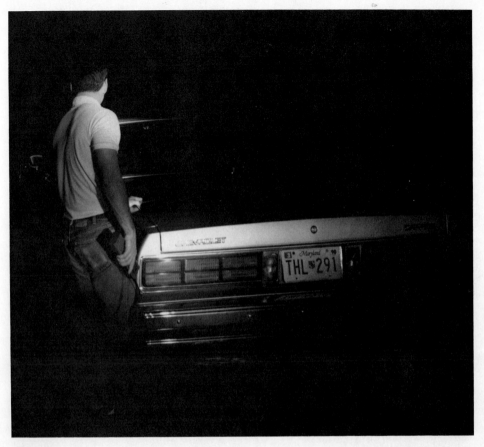

FIGURE 2-5
When the unit is properly positioned, the rescuer's shadow will be cast in the roadway rather than in the vehicle's mirrors.

tween the spotlight and the vehicle. This action will momentarily provide a silhouette in the vehicle's rearview mirror and alert the occupants to your exact position. Strategic use of lighting is essential to the element of surprise.

Each rescuer should take a flashlight when leaving the unit, but the light should remain off until the approach is complete and a need to see inside of the vehicle exists.

When leaving the unit, always remember to carry a pad of paper to record vital signs and other pertinent patient information. Many rescuers carry a small pad of paper in their shirt pocket whenever on duty. The pad should be carried in the left hand when making all of the approaches discussed in Chapter 3. Use of the pad as a distraction technique will be discussed in Chapter 4.

▼   **SURVIVAL TIPS**   ▼

1 Most vehicles are equipped with a door-activated switch that automatically turns on the interior lights when a door is opened. Disconnect this switch to prevent lighting the interior of the unit. After the scene is found to be safe, the interior light may be activated with the manual dash switch.

2 If the occupants of a vehicle approached at night adjust their mirrors to prevent the lights that have been directed on them from reflecting inside of their vehicle, you should recognize a potentially dangerous situation. Request law enforcement to investigate the situation. Withdraw the rescue unit to a safe area and await the arrival of the police.

3

APPROACHING THE MOTOR VEHICLE

Many law enforcement personnel killed in the line of duty each year are fatally wounded after leaving the relative safety of the patrol car to approach a stopped vehicle. Over the years, law enforcement agencies have devised and refined various techniques that allow personnel to approach a stopped vehicle safely.

In recent years, individually developed approach skills have been assembled into a system for responders to use when approaching a stopped vehicle. When used properly, this mental checklist gives the responder a maximum degree of safety.

These systems are not usually needed on incidents such as personal-injury accidents at a busy intersection, accidents where the vehicle is found torn wide open, or situations with bystanders already around the vehicle. These are the easy ones; they are the calls that we have been most thoroughly trained to handle, and they present a minimal amount of danger to the rescuer's personal safety.

An approach system may be most beneficial in those incidents where something you sense on arrival gives you a very uncomfortable feeling about approaching the vehicle. This simple and systematic procedure is easily adaptable for use by all emergency services personnel.

After the emergency response unit is properly positioned and all preparations to be completed before leaving the vehicle (see Chapter 2) are accomplished, the approach may begin. When the unit is carrying two or more responders, the person riding in the right front seat of the emergency vehicle makes the approach. This person is usually the officer in charge

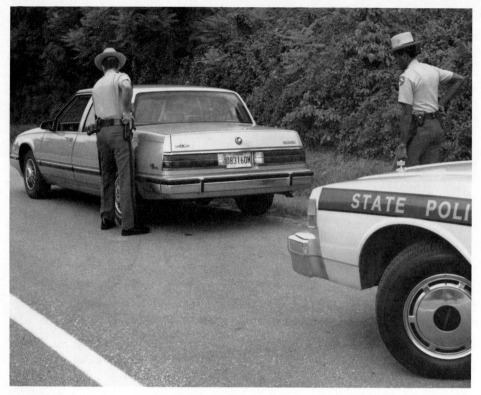

FIGURE 3-1
The police officers approaching this automobile are prepared to use force to
control the situation.

(OIC) of the emergency vehicle and the most experienced member of the
crew.

Many law enforcement agencies use two officers when approaching a
stopped vehicle (Figure 3-1). If one of the advancing officers is attacked, the
other officer has the ability to use deadly force if necessary to neutralize
the situation. Firefighting and emergency medical service agencies are not
equipped with the necessary weapons to deal with this type of incident.
Use of the single person approach procedure ensures that only one person
is placed in a possibly dangerous situation. All other members of the emergency response team remain with the medic unit or engine company in case
something goes wrong.

DRIVER-SIDE APPROACH

Anyone who has been stopped for a moving violation knows that the
law enforcement officer usually walks up to the driver's side of the vehicle
and asks for a driver's license and registration. This method of approach is

so common that the driver is often holding the license and registration out the window by the time the officer reaches the side of the car. This is the most common method of approach and has been used by law enforcement personnel for many years.

What is not usually recognized by the general public is the systematic method in which the officer moves from the patrol car to the side of the stopped vehicle. All emergency services personnel should become proficient in making this approach.

The approach begins when you, as the OIC, get out of the right side of the unit. Close the door quietly to maintain the element of surprise. If the door is slammed shut, the occupants of the vehicle will know by the noise that someone has left the unit. The closed door will also permit the driver to move the unit quickly, if necessary. Remove only the jump kit (aid bag) from the unit for the initial approach.

Do not take the electrocardiogram (ECG) monitor, oxygen, and other gear to the scene unless there is an obvious emergency. An excessive amount of equipment may interfere with your ability to move quickly. At this time you are the *only* person to leave the unit and approach the vehicle. Until you determine that the scene is safe, all other personnel should remain in the unit.

After leaving the unit, walk around the rear of the unit, continue walking forward on the driver's side, and stop at the driver's door (Figure 3-2). Because the situation could change while you are out of sight of the other vehicle, move around the rear of the unit as quickly as possible. If you arrive on the scene alone, start the approach from the driver-side door. You do not have to pass around the rear of the unit.

If you are assigned to a busy company, you do not always feel like walking all the way around the unit. In fact, you may not feel like doing any more work than is absolutely necessary. No matter how tired you may be, make it a habit to walk behind the unit instead of walking between the two vehicles. Some examples of why you should not walk between the vehicles include the following:

- ▸ At night, you will be silhouetted by the headlights of your own unit when you walk between the two vehicles. The occupants of the vehicle will know exactly where you are, and the element of surprise is lost.
- ▸ If your vehicle is struck from behind, you may be crushed between the unit and the stopped vehicle.
- ▸ While you are between the vehicles, the driver of the stopped vehicle may accidentally shift into reverse instead of park, which may make the vehicle lurch backward.
- ▸ The person in the other vehicle may be wanted by the police. The driver may intentionally shift into reverse to injure you, which will give ample time to escape in the ensuing confusion.

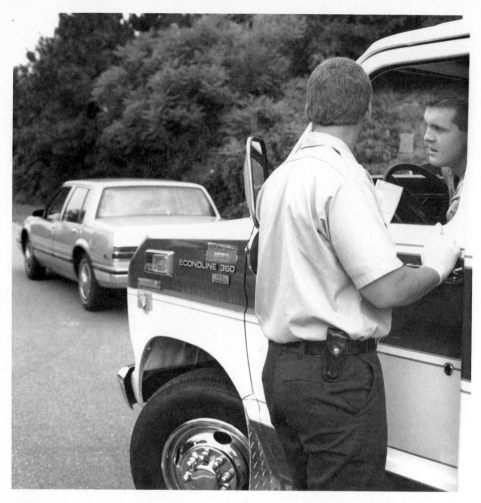

FIGURE 3-2
Before approaching the stopped vehicle, the officer in charge walks around the unit and stops at the unit driver's door.

▶ If either vehicle accidentally rolls toward the other, you may be crushed in between.

When you reach the unit driver's door, discuss any changes in the overall situation. While you are walking around the unit, the emergency vehicle driver's responsibility is to observe the occupants of the vehicle in front. If either you or the driver have noticed any signs of danger, the approach must stop, and law enforcement assistance should be requested. Danger signals include the driver of the vehicle in front positioning the mirror to view your approach or heads popping up from the back seat and then disappearing. When you decide to abort the approach, the unit's driver should back the unit a safe distance away from the other vehicle and

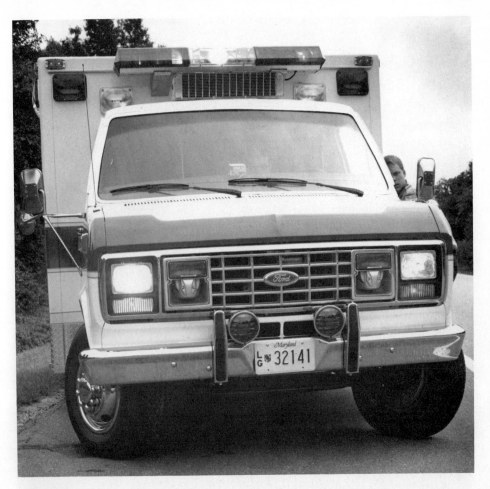

FIGURE 3-3
The OIC is protected by the front left fender and front left wheel, which can stop a
.357 Magnum. When crouched close to the floor, the driver is protected by the
engine block.

call for help. Until law enforcement personnel arrive and declare the vehicle safe, all emergency services personnel should remain in a protected
area (Figure 3-3).

As you continue the approach, you will enter the open area between
the front of the unit and the rear of the car. Very little can be done for protection in this area. Make this portion of the approach quietly and quickly.
Lift your feet when walking; do not kick the gravel. Try to prevent keys or
pocket change from jingling.

Move directly from the left front fender of the unit to the rear driver-
side trunk area of the vehicle. Quietly put the jump kit on the ground near
the back of the vehicle's trunk. Place the jump kit where you will not trip

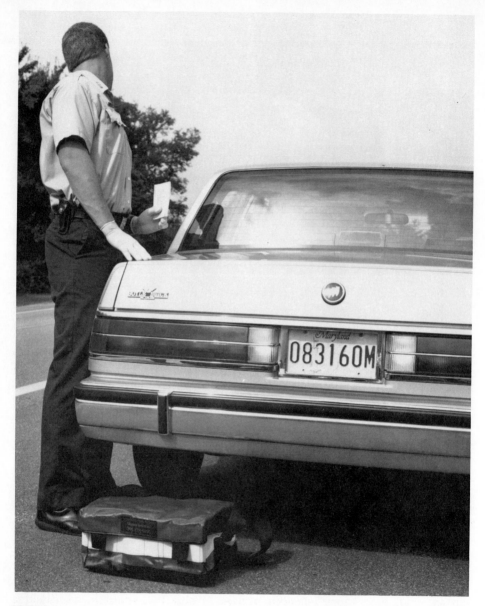

FIGURE 3-4
If the situation goes out of control and your life is endangered, do not stop to pick up the jump kit.

over it should a hurried retreat become necessary. Place your right hand lightly on the seam between the trunk lid and the left quarter panel (Figure 3-4) and check for any evidence that the trunk lid is not secure. Hand placement should be light enough not to move the vehicle. If the trunk lid feels abnormally higher than the left quarter panel, the lid may not be latched

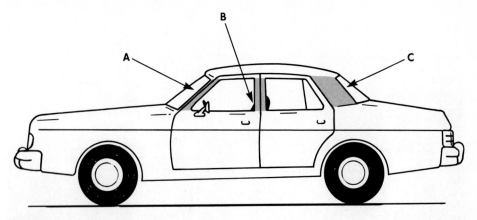

FIGURE 3-5
"A," "B," and "C" columns of a vehicle.

and someone may be hiding in the trunk. If the lid is ajar or movement is felt in the trunk, slam the lid to prevent the occupant from exiting the trunk. Do *not* lift the trunk lid to slam it shut—push it down instead. If you lift the lid and then slam it, you have lost the element of surprise. Occupants of the vehicle would know exactly where you are and that you are suspicious of the situation. If this happens, your life is suddenly in danger, and you are no longer in control of the situation.

Avoid the area near the trunk lock. An armed occupant in a trunk may fire through the vehicle and try to hit anyone thought to be preparing to insert a key in the lock.

A "click" may indicate the trunk has been unlocked from inside the vehicle. If you hear this click, immediately abort the approach and retreat to a safe location. To learn to recognize this sound, stand near the rear of a vehicle while a friend unlocks the trunk from inside the vehicle.

In the fall of 1972, officers from the Montgomery County Police Department in Maryland arrested the only apparent occupant of a vehicle. He and another man were wanted for the armed robbery of a shoe store in the area. The car was impounded and towed to the Silver Spring Police Station for processing. During the investigation, officers found it difficult to gain access to the trunk of the vehicle. While attempting entry through the back seat, a police lieutenant was shot in the forehead by the second robber who had hidden in the trunk.[1] If you do not develop and follow a systematic procedure that includes checking the trunk lid, you may be the paramedic, emergency medical technician, or firefighter who is killed or wounded in a similar situation.

After ensuring that the trunk lid is secure, observe the side-view mirror. If the mirror is moving or appears to be at a strange angle, ask yourself, "Why?" If you are satisfied with the answer, move forward on the driver's side of the vehicle and stop at the "C" column (Figure 3-5). Moving

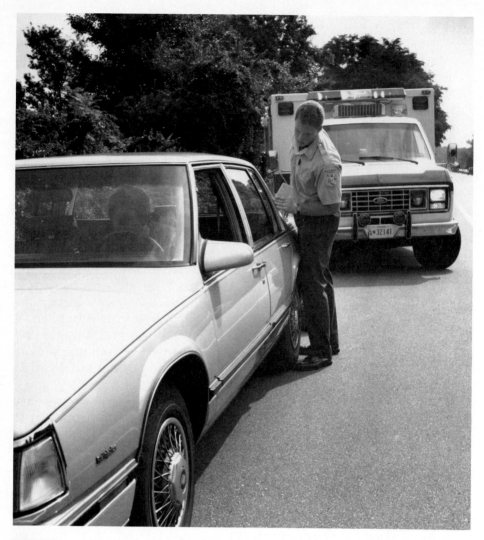

FIGURE 3-6
Stop at the left "C" column and look in the rear and side windows. Until the OIC declares the vehicle safe, the jump kit remains on the ground at the rear of the vehicle.

belly-in toward the vehicle creates as small an image as possible for the occupants of the vehicle to see and keeps you out of the flow of traffic. Anyone who has worked a highway incident knows that some motorists do not slow down for any reason. If you are standing away from the side of the vehicle, you may be hit by passing traffic.

Some irresponsible truck drivers play a game called "dusting a trooper." Spotting a trooper standing next to a stopped vehicle, the truck driver maneuvers the truck as close as possible to the side of the road and

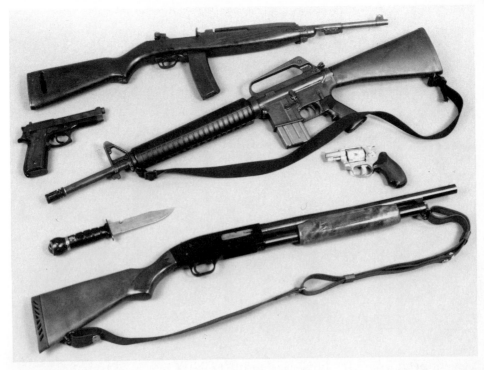

FIGURE 3-7
The primary purpose of high-threat weapons is to kill.

tries to make air rushing from the side of the passing tractor-trailer blow the trooper's hat off. Just because you are not a trooper does not mean that this could not happen to you.

Always stand sideways to the vehicle and stay as close to the vehicle as possible. You will then have maximum protection from the occupants of the vehicle and from irresponsible motorists that pass.

Stop at the left "C" column and look in the rear and side windows (Figure 3-6). Notice the number of people in the vehicle. Pay particular attention to the location of their hands. Try to see what items are lying on the seat or on the floor. Look for weapons. If a high-threat weapon such as a gun or knife is observed (Figure 3-7), abort the approach, retreat to a protected area, and call for police assistance. Once the approach has been aborted, do not resume the approach until law enforcement personnel arrive on the scene and declare the vehicle safe.

The presence of low-threat weapons should heighten your awareness of potential danger. Unless an indication that the occupants of the vehicle intend to use the weapons against you exists, do not abort the approach. Anything that can be used as a weapon not in the high-threat weapon category is considered a low-threat weapon (Figure 3-8). Innumerable items

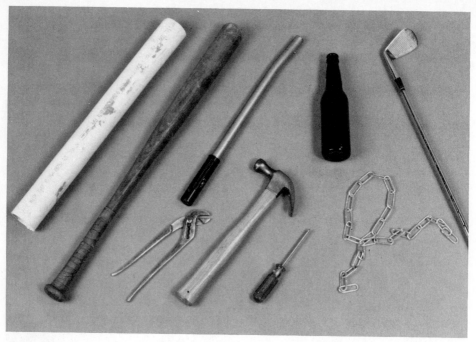

FIGURE 3-8
Low-threat weapons can also be used to kill; however, this is not their primary purpose.

normally found inside a vehicle can be considered low-threat weapons. You can do nothing about these items, but you need to be aware of their presence in case the occupant makes a sudden move toward one. If a move is made, recognize the unexpected threat and immediately retreat to a protected area. Follow the same procedures for an aborted approach in this situation as you do for high-threat weapons.

If the back seat is occupied, do not pass the "C" column. Passing the "C" column will place the back-seat passengers behind you. You have to divide your attention between the front and rear seats, which places you in an unfavorable position. When working an incident, treat rear-seat passengers and anyone standing behind you as potential threats. Exercise caution any time a civilian is standing behind you.

After observing no passengers in the back seat or any visible high-threat weapons, move forward to the "B" column with the same belly-in movement. As with the "C" column, the "B" column will conceal you from the passengers of the vehicle. Before attempting aggressive action, a driver posing a threat would have to turn in the seat, see you, and focus on you. As long as you remain behind the "B" column, you should have time to retreat to a safe area. Do *not* proceed to the driver's door at this time (Figure 3-9). The front seat checklist must still be carried out. Ask yourself, "Where

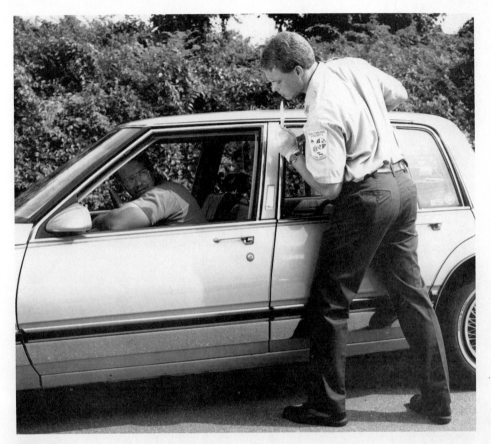

FIGURE 3-9
At this stage of the approach, do *not* move past the "B" column for any reason!

are the occupants' hands? What are the occupants doing? Are any weapons visible?"

The front-seat area of a vehicle provides many places to conceal a weapon. These locations include the following:

- ▶ On top of the sun visor
- ▶ Under either side of the seat
- ▶ In the glove box
- ▶ In side-door pockets
- ▶ In the center console
- ▶ Between bucket seats
- ▶ Next to the driver's right thigh

Be especially alert to the possibility of a gun next to the driver's right thigh. Since the driver is the person usually in charge of a civilian vehicle, anyone approaching a stopped vehicle is expected to walk to the driver's

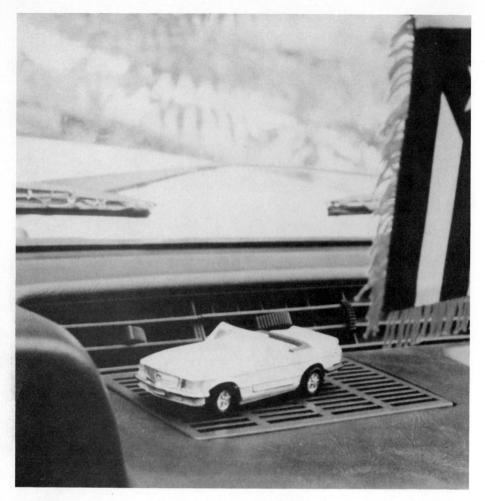

FIGURE 3-10
Grill in place. *(Courtesy Colin Perkins, Bath Police Department, Akron, Ohio.)*

door. If you approach the vehicle as expected, you will not see a weapon next to the driver's thigh. Watch the occupants' hands; their direction of movement may give away the location of an unseen weapon. The innocent-looking model car attached to the dashboard speaker grill in Figure 3-10 can serve as a handle to remove the grill for quick access to the two semi-automatic weapons and extra ammunition concealed in the void space under the grill (Figure 3-11).

When you are ready to let the driver know that you are there, do so without moving past the "B" column into the driver-door area. Law enforcement personnel refer to this area as the *kill zone.* Dangerous situations in this area include the following:

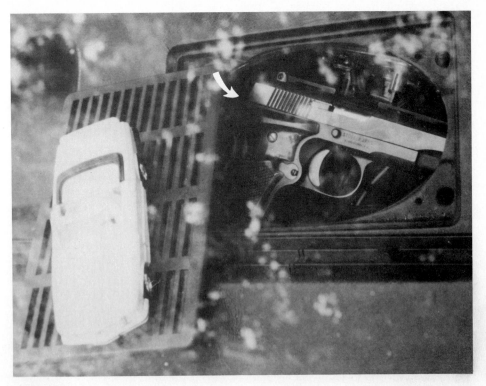

FIGURE 3-11
Grill removed. *(Courtesy Colin Perkins, Bath Police Department, Akron, Ohio.)*

- The driver can push the door open and knock you off-balance. If this happens, you have lost control of the situation and your life is in danger.
- A .22 caliber bullet is capable of passing through a car door. If a handgun is lying on the driver's lap, all the person has to do is pull the trigger when you reach the driver's door. Then you become part of the problem.
- If you pass the "C" column with the back seat occupied, the same threats are posed.

Tap lightly on the window of the vehicle to get the driver's attention and announce yourself: "Pikesville Fire Company, do you need assistance?" There can be no doubt that you are from the fire department, paramedic, or ambulance service. Make it clear that you are there to help the patient. You may be mistaken for a police officer.

Do not reach inside the car for any reason. The driver can grab your arm and pull you into the car or against the roof. This situation may result in your injury or death. Conducting the primary survey concealed by the "B"

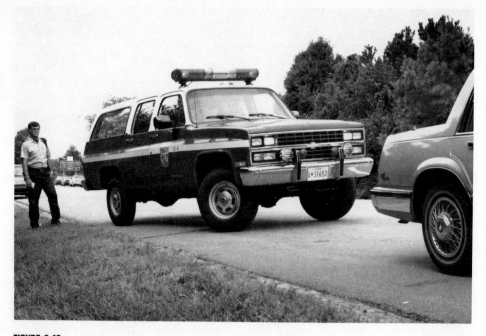

FIGURE 3-12
The passenger-side approach requires the person who has responded alone to exit from the driver's door and walk around the rear of the unit.

column is safer. Once you determine that the driver needs medical care, check that the vehicle is in park and signal for the medic unit driver to move forward with the additional equipment.

After the officer in charge declares the incident scene safe and the determination is made that medical or other assistance is required by the occupants of the vehicle, all personnel on the scene will follow the standard operating procedures for their department.

PASSENGER-SIDE APPROACH

Approaching the vehicle from the passenger side enhances your element of surprise and therefore increases your odds of survival if violence erupts.

After you complete the necessary preparations in the unit (see Chapter 2), the approach to the vehicle begins. The OIC is again responsible for making the approach, but in this example the approach will be along the passenger side of the vehicle.

The occupants of the vehicle will expect you to approach the driver's side of the vehicle. The driver is usually looking in the mirror for you to make the usual approach, and they are waiting for you. If you systematically approach the vehicle from the passenger side, the occupants of the vehicle will be surprised when they see you, and you may be surprised at what you see.

A Maryland State Police trooper made a night stop of a vehicle and carried out all of the systematic checks during the approach from the passenger side. As the driver was watching through the side mirror for the approaching trooper, the officer stood by the right "B" column watching the driver stuff bags of marijuana under the front seat.[2] When the trooper tapped on the right-side window, the driver turned with an "I'm caught" look and started removing the bags from under the seat. If the approach had been from the driver's side of the vehicle, the trooper would not have seen this movement; it could have been a weapon instead of bags being concealed.

In single-person response units the driver must exit from the driver's door and walk around the rear of the unit as the OIC did in the first approach discussed (Figure 3-12). For units responding with more than one person, you (the OIC) exit from the passenger door with the jump kit and proceed quickly and quietly to the trunk on the passenger side. Ensure that your unit is properly parked on a 10-degree angle with the wheels cut to the left (see Chapter 2). Remember, as soon as you step out of the unit you are completely exposed. No protection from the unit exists as in the driver's side approach. Do not hesitate after exiting the unit. Proceed directly to the rear passenger–side trunk area and place the jump kit at the rear of the vehicle out of the path of travel (Figure 3-13).

Check the trunk lid in the same manner. Remember to use only a light touch on the trunk seam to detect motion or an unsecured trunk lid.

Using the same belly-in movement, proceed to the "C" column on the passenger side of the vehicle. Make the same checks for high- and low-threat weapons, and observe the occupants of the back seat. What are they doing? Where are their hands?

After you find that the back seat is safe, continue to the "B" column. Keep your belly in toward the vehicle. Check for high- and low-threat weapons. How many people are in the front seat? Where are their hands? While you check the front-seat area, use the "B" column for concealment and protection.

Stay out of the kill zone. Remember that the person in the passenger seat can give you the same problems as the driver being approached on the driver's side. If you are standing in the kill zone, either the passenger or the driver has a straight shot at you when they turn to acknowledge your presence.

Recognize that most weapons are hidden from personnel expected to approach on the driver's side of the vehicle. When standing on the passenger side, you are in the best possible position to observe any device that could be aggressively used against you, but you must stay behind the "B" column.

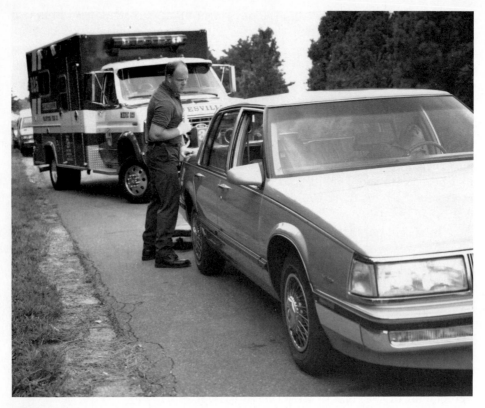

FIGURE 3-13
Officer in charge moves from the right-front door of the unit directly to the right
rear–trunk area of the vehicle.

After determining that the vehicle and the occupants are not a threat,
announce your presence in a similar manner as described for the driver-
side approach. Complete the primary survey and notify your partner to approach the vehicle. Your partner can bring any additional equipment that
may be needed.

Law enforcement agencies, emergency medical services, and fire departments that use both the driver-side approach and the passenger-side
approach claim that a greater margin of safety is available to personnel
that use the passenger-side approach. Several of the reasons for this claim
include the following:

- The person making the approach is out of the flow of traffic.
- A greater variety of cover is available to the person making the approach.
- The distance between the person making the approach and the
  driver of the stopped vehicle is greater, which allows the emergency
  services worker more time to react to an adverse situation.

▶ The interior design of most automobiles does not allow for quick movements to the right. For example, the driver cannot point a gun at a person standing behind the "B" column without moving over the seats or the head rest.

In the author's experience the driver-side approach should be made during daylight hours. The occupants of the stopped vehicle can watch you through the rearview mirrors regardless of the side of approach. The passenger-side approach has the greatest advantage during low-light conditions and at night with heavy shadows and strong lights providing protection for a high-risk approach.

Be prepared for the occupant(s) of the vehicle to be uncomfortable with your approach on the passenger side. The driver may ask, "What are you doing over there?" or insist that you "Come around to this side!" Your response should be, "Well, sir, I would prefer to work from this side. Please open the passenger side door for me." If this happens, you will know that your approach from the passenger side has put the occupant(s) off-balance. Use this information to your advantage. Take control of the situation. Let the occupant(s) know, in a professional manner, that you are in charge. Stay on the passenger side.

VARIATION FOR VANS

Historically, van stops have been the most dangerous traffic stop for law enforcement officers. A van may be occupied by a single person driving or contain as many as 15 people that cannot be seen (Figure 3-14). Vans can carry virtually any type of cargo, and the inability to visualize that cargo makes an approach to a van dangerous for fire department and emergency medical services personnel. During a gasoline shortage, an Ohio man installed a 275-gallon fuel tank in his van to transport stolen gasoline (Figure 3-15).[3] Consider the hazard this vehicle presents to the emergency services if it is involved in a traffic accident with people trapped inside or if the van is involved in a fire.

Vans are known to transport arms used by both motorcycle gangs and terrorist groups. Whenever a motorcycle gang is moving over the road in formation, at least one van is usually close behind, operated by gang members to carry the gang's weapons. Large-caliber machine guns mounted for firing out of the rear doors of vans are also a possibility.

When approaching a van incident, exercise extreme caution. Because there are too many doors to watch simultaneously, the opportunity for one or more passengers to exit and come up behind you is a danger.

When a van is involved, the driver-side approach is *not* recommended. Since the emergency services worker makes the approach on the opposite side of the van from the sliding door, you may think it would be the safer side. It is not—this is the expected approach, and the occupants will anticipate your position.

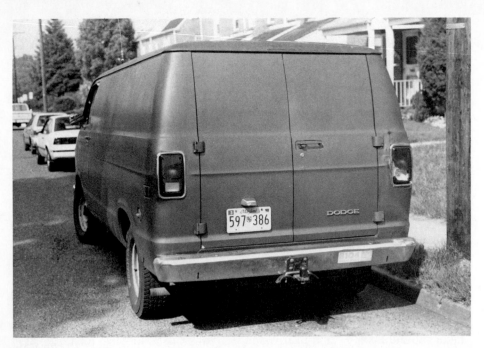

FIGURE 3-14
Vans are capable of carrying large numbers of people, contraband, and hazardous cargo.

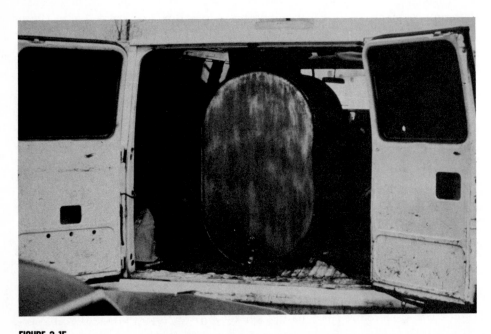

FIGURE 3-15
Fuel tank installed to transport gasoline illegally. *(Courtesy William S. Ennis, Sr., West Carrollton Division of Fire, West Carrollton, Ohio.)*

When using the driver-side approach on a van, you give up the element of surprise, since there is no "C" column to pause behind while checking the rear of the vehicle for weapons and occupants. The first contact with the occupants, by necessity of construction, is not until you reach the "B" column. Because of the height of the door window, you will probably be unable to see the front seat area from this position. You cannot see a passenger in the right front seat without stepping in front of the "B" column and placing yourself in the kill zone.

On 10 August 1975, a Maryland State Police sergeant stopped a van on the eastern shore of Maryland. The van matched the description of one suspected of carrying armed robbery suspects. The sergeant positioned the cruiser at the "B" column of the van and was talking door-to-door with the van driver. An unseen occupant sitting behind the driver placed a shotgun against the inside of the sheet-metal van, pulled the trigger, and killed the sergeant. The passenger who did the shooting did not have to see the target. The killer knew exactly where the trooper was going to stop.

All van approaches should be made from the passenger side. Preparations for the approach are the same as the approaches described in Chapter 2. As part of the preparation before leaving the unit, discuss with the unit driver the rear doors of the van. Do not physically check the rear doors as you would a trunk lid. Agree on the condition of the doors (latched, unlatched), and agree on an audible warning signal that the unit driver will sound if the position of the rear doors or the driver's door changes during the approach.

The actual approach is modified from the passenger-side approach discussed. When approaching a van, do not move forward on the side of the van or use the belly-in method recommended for the other approaches. In this position an occupant may suddenly open the side door and grab you.

In van incidents, you may get your shoes dirty. When you exit the unit with the jump kit, move away from the passenger side of the van to a distance of between 10 and 15 feet. If you are required to jump a guard rail or walk in a ditch, do so. Remain clear of the side door of the van throughout the approach (Figure 3-16). When this position is reached, walk parallel to the van until you reach a position approximately 45-degrees forward of the "A" column.

The position shown in Figure 3-17 allows the greatest visibility inside of the van but maintains a safe distance until the situation is determined to be secure. The occupants are not going to expect you to be in this position. By maintaining the element of surprise, you effectively control the situation.

From this point, you can announce your presence. Identify yourself as "Fire Department" or "Emergency Medical Services" and ask, "Did you call for an ambulance?" If the answers are to your satisfaction and medical assistance is required, call for the rest of the crew to meet you at the van and begin treatment according to your standard operating procedures.

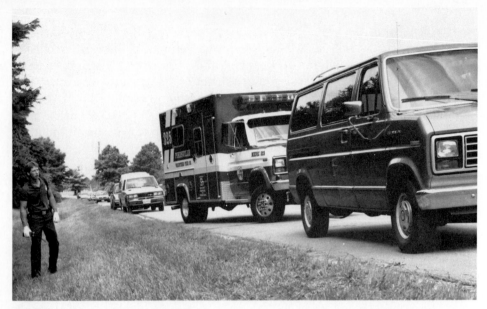

FIGURE 3-16
Until you are 45-degrees forward of the "A" column, maintain 10 to 15 feet between yourself and the passenger side of the van.

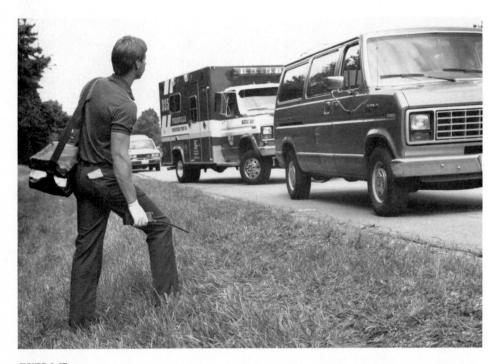

FIGURE 3-17
Position yourself 45-degrees forward of the "A" column before making contact with the occupants of a van.

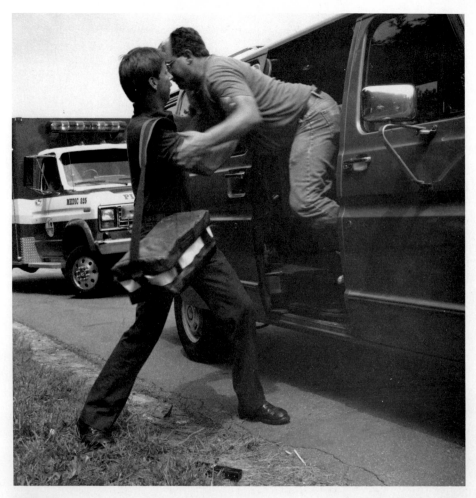

FIGURE 3-18
The area near the side door is known as the *grab area*. Attempting to flee through this area increases your chance of being injured.

If no response is given to your calls, no one is visible from your position, and no indications that this is other than a normal incident are observed, move quietly to the "A" column and look on the floor of the van. The patient may be lying there in cardiac arrest.

If you have to flee the van from your position near the "A" column because of aggressive action from the occupants, you may have to seek cover away from the emergency response unit (see Chapter 9). Do not run directly to the emergency response unit from a position near the front of the van. If you do, you will pass near the side door of the van and increase your chance of being attacked (Figure 3-18).

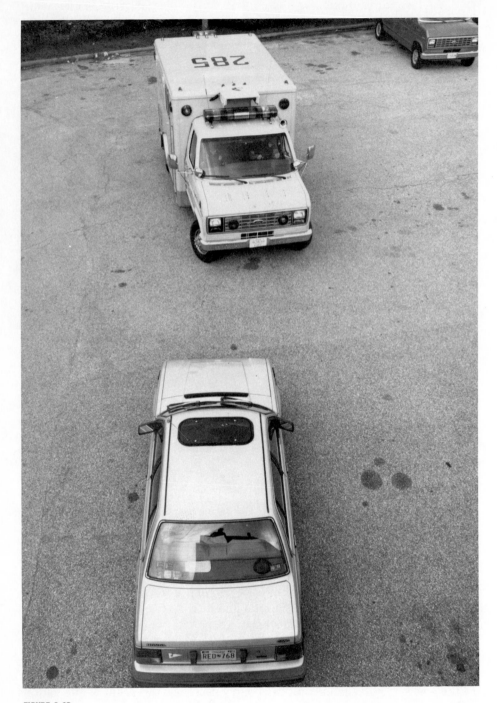

FIGURE 3-19
Not all approaches are made to the rear.

When visibility inside any vehicle is obscured by foggy or tinted windows, use the variation for vans approach. Usually the windshield is clearer than the other windows and is the most useful for scanning the interior of the vehicle.

THE HEAD-ON APPROACH

In some circumstances, positioning the emergency response unit at the rear of the vehicle in question is not practical; for example, when you approach the scene from the opposite direction of travel or when the vehicle is located on a parking lot (Figure 3-19). When this situation occurs, if you continue past the vehicle to turn around and approach from the rear, you have lost the element of surprise. In these situations, use the head-on approach.

This approach requires the emergency response driver to stop the unit approximately 15 feet from the front of the vehicle on a 10-degree angle to the unit driver's left. If the call is a night response, place headlights on high-beam and aim any spotlights through the vehicle's windshield to conceal your exit from the unit. All other preparations for leaving the unit have been previously described in Chapter 2.

Exit the unit with the jump kit, walk around the rear of the unit, and stop at the driver's door for updated information on activity in or around the vehicle. After determining the safety of the approach, move away from the passenger side of the vehicle for a distance of 10 to 15 feet. Walk parallel to the vehicle until you reach a position approximately 45 degrees behind the vehicle. From this position move directly to the right rear trunk section of the vehicle, place the jump kit on the ground, and proceed with a normal passenger-side approach (Figure 3-20).

This modified passenger-side approach is recommended for day and night responses that require a head-on arrival at the scene. While attempting to reach the recommended position at the "B" column of the vehicle, the rescuer using this approach can remain clear of the kill zone.

TIME FRAME FOR STARTING TREATMENT

When arriving on a scene, pause momentarily to assess your surroundings before starting patient treatment. After ensuring your personal safety, make a systematic approach to the vehicle in a timely manner, recognize the occupant's problem(s), and initiate basic and advanced life support consistent with accepted practices.

You may be questioned by your superiors, the press, the victim, or the victim's relatives or attorneys about why you took these precautions before starting treatment. Your best defense is that you were making sure the scene was safe for you to get to the vehicle and assist the patient without jeopardizing yourself. The Department of Transportation (DOT) National

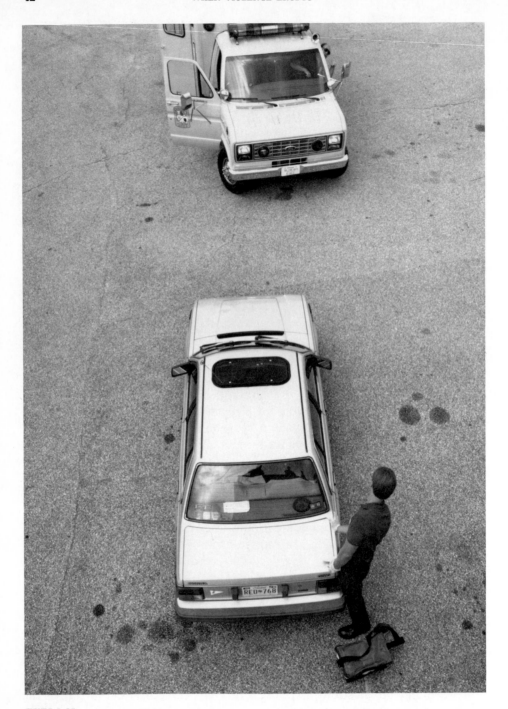

FIGURE 3-20
Until you are 45-degrees behind the vehicle, maintain 10 to 15 feet between
yourself and the passenger side of the vehicle. Once you reach this position,
proceed with a normal passenger-side approach.

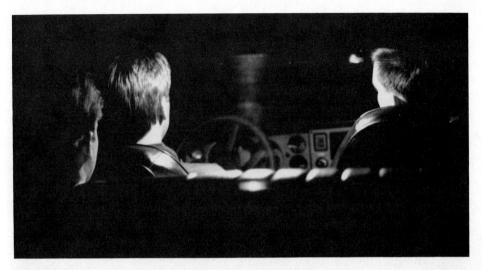

FIGURE 3-21
Before starting a night approach, direct the occupants of the vehicle to turn on the interior light.

Standard Curriculum for EMT requires a check for scene safety as part of the primary survey.

The methods of approach described in this chapter may appear to require an unacceptable amount of time to complete. However, with proper training and practice the approach should be completed and treatment started within 30 to 45 seconds after you leave the unit.

▼　　　　　　　**SURVIVAL TIPS**　　　　　　　▼

1　Incidents occur where you should not approach a vehicle until a law enforcement unit arrives on the scene, for example, when people are holding weapons or yelling and cursing at you. Other times are not so obvious. No hard and fast rules define what is a go or no-go situation. If you feel (for whatever reason) you may be in danger, *do not approach the vehicle.*

2　Your license or contract does not say that just because you are wearing an EMT, fire department, or paramedic patch you have to place yourself in danger of bodily harm. If you are uncomfortable with a situation, you can use the public address system on your unit to give instructions to the occupants of the vehicle before you leave the unit.

3　Directing occupants to turn on the interior light before starting a night approach will enhance your ability to identify how many occupants are in the vehicle, their positions in the vehicle, and any potentially hostile movements they may make during the approach (Figure 3-21). Illuminat-

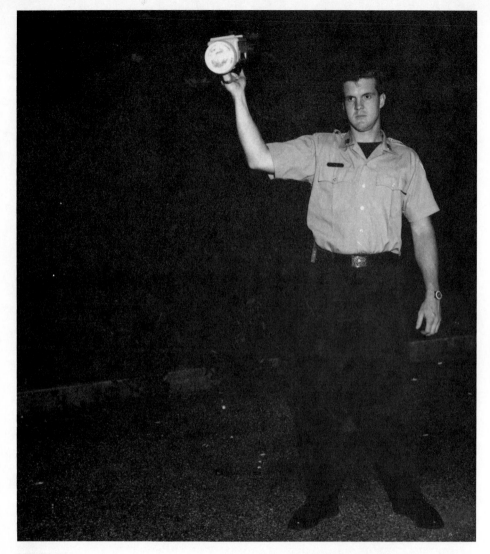

FIGURE 3-22
Because a light makes a good target, hold a flashlight away from your body when illuminating an area.

ing the interior light may also assist in concealing the approaching rescuer from the vehicle's occupants.

4   Because no one is in the unit to call for assistance, a lone responder that arrives on the scene should always take a portable radio when leaving the unit. Make sure the portable radio is on low volume before exiting the unit so that the element of surprise will not be lost because of an unexpected radio transmission from another unit on the same frequency.

5 Flashlights should remain off until needed. Hold the light at arms-length and away from the body before turning it on (Figure 3-22). Illuminate the scene for only a few seconds during each use.

6 When all four doors of the vehicle open and all of the occupants start walking toward the emergency response unit, use the public address system. Tell them to return to their vehicle. The scene is easier to control when the occupants remain inside of the vehicle rather than outside wandering around. If your instructions are ignored, you are still in a position to back away from the scene (see Chapter 4).

7 If you are responding in a single person response unit, create the effect of more than one rescuer approaching the vehicle (night approaches only) by slamming the door of the unit twice. If the unit has been properly positioned (see Chapter 2), the occupants of the vehicle cannot see you approaching because of the blinding lights from the unit. Reinforce this illusion by carrying on a conversation with your imaginary partner who remains unseen on the other side of the vehicle.

8 Do not become complacent—repetitive calls with no problems can have a deadly effect. Consider the need for using an approach system on each incident involving a motor vehicle.

9 Heavy armaments and armor plating may be encountered on vehicles operated by high-ranking government officials, heads of large corporations, or your local drug dealer. Optional equipment on these vehicles may include smoke grenade or tear-gas launchers located behind front and rear bumpers or in the trunk compartment.[4]

4

FLEEING AN ARMED ENCOUNTER

The medic unit arrives at the scene of a car stopped on the side of the highway for a reported "man having difficulty breathing in a motor vehicle." The only visible occupant of the vehicle (the driver) appears to have a problem breathing. When the rescuer reaches the "B" column and announces, "Woodlawn Fire Company, are you okay?" the driver turns in the seat, and a pistol becomes visible in his right hand. His intentions are to shoot the rescuers and take the drug box, hypodermic needles, and anything that may turn a quick dollar at the local crack house.

Fortunately, an occupant seated in a motor vehicle must make several moves to initiate aggressive action against a rescuer who is properly positioned to the rear of the appropriate column. If the action centers on the use of a firearm, the aggressor must do the following:

- ▶ **TURN** Physically turn in the seat, with the trunk twisted toward the rescuer
- ▶ **LOCATE** Visually locate the position of the rescuer
- ▶ **FOCUS** Focus on the rescuer to accurately take aim
- ▶ **FIRE** Point and fire the weapon

Each of these actions requires time to carry out. Your responsibility is to make the best possible use of this time and successfully avoid the intended aggression. If you can interrupt any of the above steps, your chance of surviving a shooting incident is increased.

Statistics published by the Federal Bureau of Investigation (FBI) show that most shootings are not like those depicted in television programs.[1]

47

They do not occur at 100 yards, nor are innumerable rounds fired. A shooting is a very intimate experience. Usually the participants are less than 5 feet apart, and the incident is generally over in less than 4 seconds with a total of 3 rounds fired.[2] Your chance of survival may depend on any action that delays the person with the weapon from firing, therefore increasing the time available for you to put distance between yourself and the other person.

THE ARMED PATIENT

Arriving on the scene of a personal-injury accident, you find a single vehicle against a tree. You determine the vehicle apparently missed a curve and ran off the road. The lone occupant of the vehicle is a male, approximately 35 years old, awake, but slow to respond. His soft-tissue facial injury was caused by the steering wheel and windshield and indicates the seat belt was not worn. As with so many injuries that could have been prevented or reduced, this is a classic case of a failure to buckle-up.

As the only unit on the scene, you systematically approach the vehicle, determine it is a legitimate incident, and signal your partner to join you. You announce, "Fire Department Paramedic, we're here to help you. Where do you hurt?" This announcement brings a response of several moans and some movement of the arms and upper body. As you complete the primary survey, your partner opens the driver's door, and the first thing you both notice is a 2-inch revolver stuck in the patient's waist belt—no holster, just the pistol (Figure 4-1).

Stop! Who is this guy? He is probably not a law enforcement officer because a police officer seldom carries a gun without a holster. It is an unsafe practice—the gun may go off. Also, most law enforcement officers purchase their own off-duty weapons. They want a weapon they can rely on, so they take care of it. A holster reduces the risk of the gun falling on the ground, keeps the gun clean, and keeps the gun oil from soiling clothes. In this case the person is possibly carrying the gun illegally.

In a situation where the gun is in a holster or you have that gut feeling that the individual may be a police officer, ask, "Are you on the job? What agency are you with?"

In any case a decision must be made. Do you attempt to take the gun? Do you back off and call for the police to take the gun? Or do you act as though the gun were not there and continue to treat the patient? In this example, the patient is in no immediate danger. He has a good airway and no severe bleeding. You have time to consider each option. With the patient's altered mental status, he may be too dangerous to treat safely as long as he has the weapon. Before continuing treatment, you would be well within the limits of acceptable patient care to back off to a safe distance and call for law enforcement personnel to take the gun.

If you elect to continue treatment without waiting for law enforcement

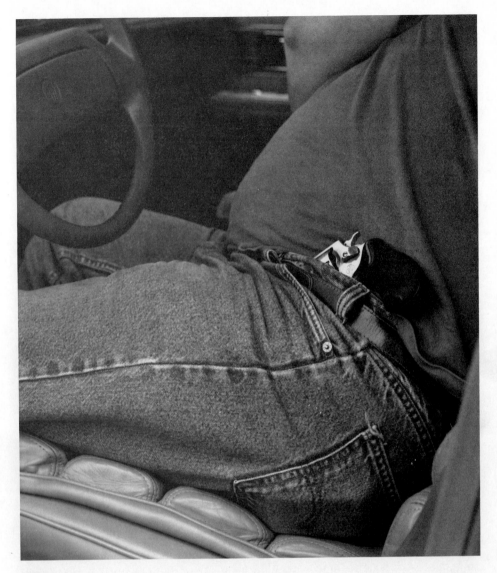

FIGURE 4-1
Because most law enforcement officers do not carry a gun unless it is in a holster, finding a gun in this position indicates a need for caution.

assistance, attempt to gather more information about the patient. As you ask the patient for identification, position yourself where you can see the gun. Ask, "Do you have any medical-assistance cards? Are you allergic to any medicines?" Check his wallet for identification. If you find a badge, ask the patient what agency employs him. Do not ask leading questions such as "Are you a cop?" which would probably result in an affirmative answer. Since you cannot be sure, tell him that you feel uncomfortable because he is armed but do not attempt to take the gun. As a result of extensive training, law enforcement officers will not surrender a weapon that may be used against them. Even though the patient is lethargic, do not attempt to remove the gun. A struggle may result, and the gun may accidentally discharge. Attempting to take the weapon exposes you, your partner, and your patient to unnecessary danger.

If the patient is unconscious or you decide to proceed with treatment as long as the patient shows no signs of aggression, immediately take the patient's radial pulse. Take the pulse on both wrists at the same time, and continue to take it until the patient is disarmed (Figure 4-2). While performing this procedure, subtly immobilize the patient's hands against the steering wheel, which should allow your partner to take the weapon safely. Depending on law enforcement personnel to arrive on the scene in time to assist in disarming the nonaggressive patient is not realistic. Because of various factors, 20 minutes or more may pass before the first police officer arrives. The courts may consider this an unnecessary delay in starting treatment.

If a weapon is in the vehicle but not physically on the person, consider moving the person away from the weapon rather than moving the weapon away from the person. After a frontal impact, objects found on the floor may have originally been on or under the seat. If a weapon is visible on the floor between or near the patient's feet, leave it there. When you touch or pick up the weapon, you become part of the chain of custody and may have to testify in court if the trial involves illegal weapons or other unlawful contents found in the vehicle.

Never leave the patient alone if a weapon is visible in the vehicle. Send someone else to get the additional equipment you need from your unit. If the patient is conscious and oriented, explain that while you are putting on the cervical collar and the short spine board (or Kendrix Extrication Device [K.E.D.] if available), you must immobilize the patient's hands and that you will release them as soon as the transfer to the medic unit is complete. At the same time, you or your partner should secure the patient's hands together with Kling dressing. Once the patient is clear of the vehicle, assign someone from the response team to secure the vehicle until law enforcement personnel arrive on the scene to accept custody of the vehicle and its contents.

If you must assume custody of a gun, write down the make and model and lock the weapon in the drug box, drug cabinet, glove box, or another secure location until the gun can be turned over to law enforcement personnel. *Never* place the weapon on the roof of the vehicle, the street, or the other end of the bench seat in the car. Do not stuff the gun into your own waist belt or back pocket. When law enforcement personnel arrive on the scene, locate the officer who is responsible for writing up the incident. Write down the name, identification or badge number of the officer, and the case number assigned to the incident before turning over custody of the

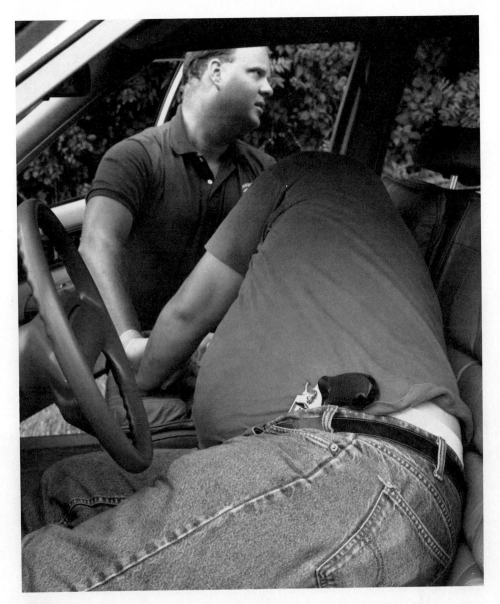

FIGURE 4-2
"I need to check your pulse and blood pressure."

weapon. Document all of this information on your run sheet and include where the weapon was found. If the patient is a law enforcement officer, treat the security of the badge with the same degree of importance as you treat the gun.

When conducting primary and secondary surveys, check for weapons while you check for injuries. Run your thumbs around the inside of a pa-

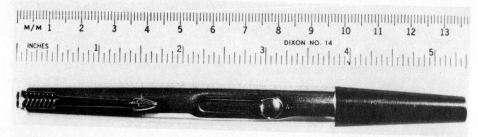

FIGURE 4-3
Many weapons do not look like weapons. This pen fires a small-caliber round.
(Courtesy Baltimore City Police Department, Baltimore.)

tient's belt to check the pelvis, spinal column, and abdominal rigidity; you may find handguns, knives, or other weapons. Do not neglect the extremities—leg and ankle holsters are very popular. If you find one weapon, look for more. Be alert for weapons that do not look like weapons: for example, a derringer attached to a belt buckle or a pen that is actually a pistol (Figure 4-3). Additional information on makeshift and concealed weapons is in Chapter 11.

If you pick up a patient from a police station or jail, never assume that a complete search has been made. As a provider of prehospital care, you must conduct a survey of your patient. Be careful because residents of these facilities may have razor blades and other small, sharp objects hidden in their cuffs, the lining of their clothes, and even in their hair.

USING THE VITALS PAD AS A DISTRACTION TECHNIQUE

While conducting drills at the Maryland State Police Glen Burnie Barracks, Trooper First Class (TFC) Raymond J. Beard successfully disrupted the chain of events in an intended shooting incident twelve out of twelve times.[3] A state police instructor sat in the driver's seat of a stopped vehicle. When asked for a driver's license, the instructor drew a weapon and squeezed the trigger in a simulation of shooting the approaching trooper. TFC Beard told the troopers participating in the exercise that if something came out of the vehicle at them, they were to take off their Stetson[4] with their left hand (driver-side approach) and throw it at the eyes of the person behind the wheel of the stopped vehicle. The intent of this action is to make the armed person blink or flinch. Throwing the hat was 100% effective—in each case the person with the weapon either misfired or misaimed.

When you drive an automobile during a heavy rain and a passing vehicle throws water on the windshield of your car, you have the same reaction. Even though you see the water coming and you know it is not going to hit you, you still blink or flinch when the water strikes the windshield. Throwing a vitals pad provides the same distraction as the water hitting

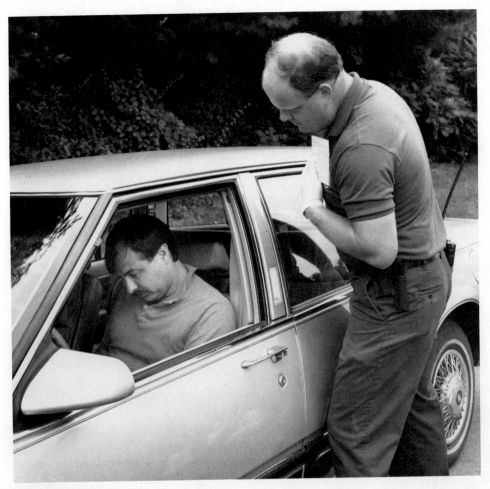

FIGURE 4-4
When conducting the initial interview, hold the vitals pad in the left hand and
raise it to the left shoulder.

the windshield or the troopers throwing their Stetsons. The chain of events
is interrupted long enough to permit the rescuer to get out of the line of fire
and run to safety.

Carry the pad in your left hand when making a driver-side approach.
When in position behind the "B" column, raise the pad to your left shoulder.
If aggressive action takes place during the initial interview with the occupant of the vehicle, be prepared to throw the pad directly at the aggressor's
nose (Figures 4-4 and 4-5). Use only a soft pad of paper for this technique. A
hard object such as an aluminum report book or clipboard may cause need-
less injuries to the occupant of the vehicle. The soft pad will not cause un-
due harm. If the vehicle's occupant is reaching for a lighter instead of a

54

WHEN VIOLENCE ERUPTS

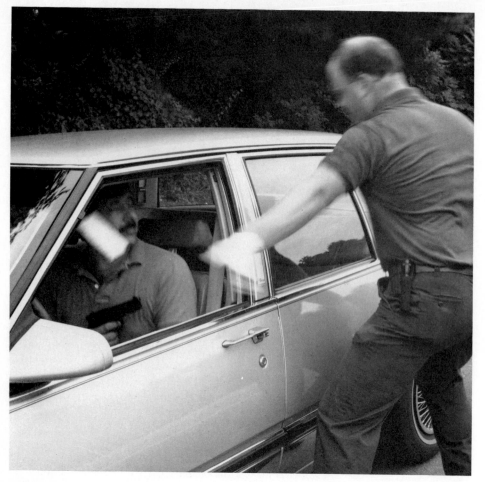

FIGURE 4-5
If aggressive action occurs, throw the pad directly at the nose of the aggressor.

weapon and you prematurely throw the vitals pad, you only have to apologize and explain. Exaggerate if necessary; say you just returned from a call where the patient took aggressive action toward you, and you thought it was going to happen again.

After the pad is thrown, do not wait for the reaction. As soon as it is out of your hand, turn to your right (toward the unit), get out of the possible line of fire, and run to safety. Do not stop and pick up the jump kit—*run!*

The object is to put as much distance as possible between you and the aggressor. If possible, run to the unit (Figure 4-6). You can call for help or drive to a safer location. If you are cut off from the unit, evaluate the surrounding area for the best possible cover and concealment (see Chapter 9).

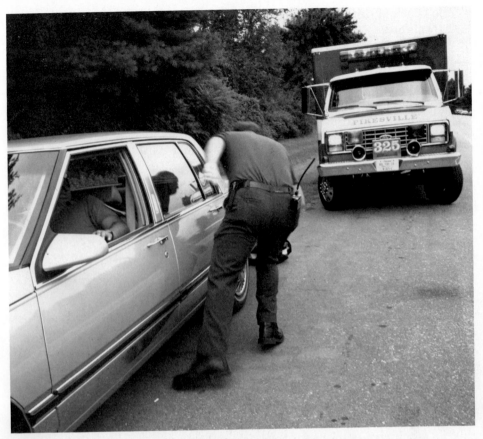

FIGURE 4-6
While the aggressor flinches and attempts to refocus, run toward the unit.

PARTNER DOWN!

As the driver of the unit, you see your partner suddenly turn from the approach with a look of panic and start to run toward the unit. After several steps, your partner falls face down in the dirt with a bullet in the back. What should you do?

Your initial reaction is to get out of the unit and run to your partner—the worst action you can take in such a situation. This decision increases the risk of no one calling for assistance because both of you are now in a dangerous and unprotected position.

The proper action is to shift into reverse and step on the accelerator. Backing away from your partner may be the toughest decision you will ever have to make, but it is the only way to increase your chances of remaining responsive long enough to call for the help that you desperately need.

Do not scream into the microphone for several seconds and then run to help your partner. If you get out of the unit, you will probably get hurt.

While waiting for the help that you hope is on the way, both of you will lie there and bleed.

Many offensive actions that avoid backing away from your partner have been suggested:

- ▶ Ramming the aggressor's vehicle
- ▶ Running down the aggressor with the unit
- ▶ Placing the unit between the aggressor and your partner

Any of these suggestions may be successful in a particular instance. However, the *best* way to assure your partner will quickly receive help is to call for all required assistance yourself. The only way to be in this position is to back away from the danger zone, remain in the unit, and provide the dispatcher with any needed information. Partners should openly discuss the possibility of this type of situation arising and agree that the uninjured partner will back off a safe distance and call for help.

BACKING AWAY FROM THE SCENE

Every emergency service response team needs a plan that describes each team member's action in a situation that has turned violent.

Certain instances require the driver of the unit to back away from the scene of a vehicle-approach:

- ▶ When high-threat weapons are observed
- ▶ When the occupants of the vehicle become unruly
- ▶ When all of the occupants exit the vehicle and approach the unit and no one appears to need emergency care
- ▶ When the area entered is a police hot zone
- ▶ When your partner has been incapacitated

Until the rescuer has completed the approach to the vehicle and assured that the scene is safe, the driver remains behind the wheel of the unit. The driver is responsible for watching the overall scene and the interior of the vehicle for any unusual activity. Anytime something looks suspicious, the driver uses a prearranged signal, such as the backup alarm, to warn the rescuer to return to the unit at once. If circumstances prevent the rescuer from immediately returning to the unit, the driver straightens the wheels of the unit and quickly backs to a safe area.

Be aware that aggressors will probably advance toward the unit as you are backing up. Statistics indicate that they usually will not follow on foot for more than 50 feet because they do not want to leave their vehicle.[5] If you have backed away for at least this distance and they continue to come toward you, back farther away. If necessary, continue backing up until the aggressors return to their vehicle. Remain at a safe distance until help arrives or the aggressors leave the scene. Backing the unit to safety gives the driver a constant view of the overall scene, moves the unit out of

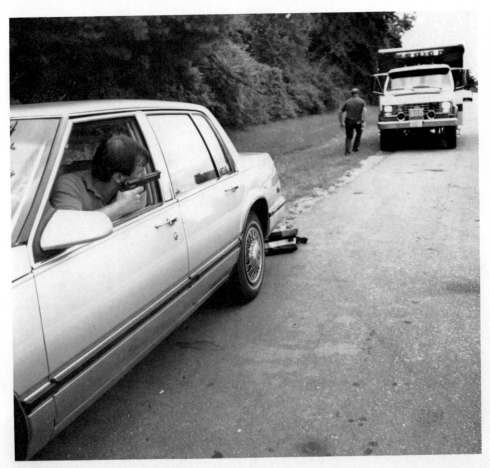

FIGURE 4-7
Backing away from the scene gives the responders the advantages of time and distance.

the danger zone, and makes a call for assistance possible (Figure 4-7).

Avoid driving forward to escape a dangerous situation because of the following reasons:

- ▶ Driving forward momentarily places the unit in the kill zone when it passes the stopped vehicle. The occupants of the vehicle have already attempted aggressive action against you. Driving forward gives them a second opportunity to harm you.
- ▶ The occupants of the stopped vehicle can follow you.
- ▶ Attempting to pull out into the flow of traffic may slow or even stop your forward motion.

When the rescuer leaves the unit, close the right-side door. If the door remains open, the side mirror will be out of position and the driver will

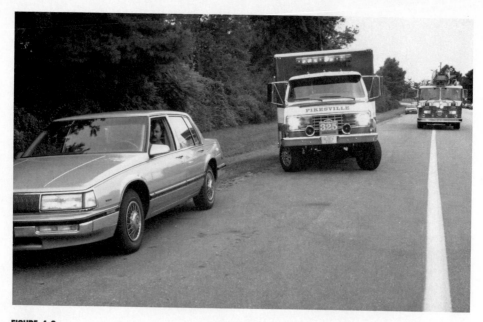

FIGURE 4-8
All responding units must understand the purpose of unit-positioning and leave
room for the first unit to retreat.

lose rear visibility on the right side of the unit. The closed door adds to the
time it takes the rescuer to get back in the unit. However, the driver can
back up the unit as soon as the rescuer begins a hasty retreat.

On incidents with two or more units responding, consider the placement of those units arriving on the scene after the first unit. If the second
unit parks immediately behind the first, the route of escape for the first
unit is blocked. The rescuers of the first unit must then modify their retreat. One solution is for them to get out of the first unit, run past the second unit, and use the latter for protection. The better solution is for all
other arriving units to remain a minimum of 50 feet to the rear of the first
unit (Figure 4-8).

JUSTIFICATIONS FOR BACKING AWAY

Backing away from a dangerous situation is not the same as leaving
the scene. Back a safe distance away from the perceived threat, call for law
enforcement assistance, and wait at that location until the scene is declared safe for you to begin or continue treatment. You must not leave the
scene until you *know* all occupants of the vehicle require no further medical treatment.

Anytime you back away from a scene, obtain a report from the law enforcement agency having jurisdiction over the area where the incident oc-

curred. Any incident involving aggressive action against the emergency service responders (no matter how minor the threat or how successful the intended aggression) requires a report. Preferring charges against the aggressor is not essential, but the police report provides critical backup documentation on an incident if the patient takes legal action at a later date. The report must clearly explain why you backed away from the area and include any acts of physical or verbal aggression carried out against you. Note in the report that you felt uncomfortable with the situation, so you backed off in self-defense to wait for law enforcement assistance.

CALLING FOR ASSISTANCE

The person calling for assistance in a time of emergency must remain calm and professional throughout the entire exchange of information. Transmissions must be clear, concise, and complete. The dispatcher will ask for the "Nature of request for police?" and then repeat everything that you have said. If your partner is down, do not worry about using the proper code. In most emergency services communications the use of plain language is far better than code. Tell the dispatcher, "My partner has just been shot, send the police!" Be ready to provide additional information.

Properly trained personnel may save time in an extreme emergency by transmitting "Signal 13," the universal law enforcement code for "officer down." This code is used *only* if personnel are in mortal danger. Until all personnel have been thoroughly indoctrinated in when to use the code, Signal 13 should not be incorporated into a department's codes and signals. Before expecting an automatic response to this code, your department must establish interagency cooperation with the law enforcement community. Without the training of all fire department and emergency medical services field personnel and dispatchers and an interagency agreement with the law enforcement community, transmitting a Signal 13 may elicit one or both of the following ineffectual responses:

- ▶ The fire department or emergency medical services dispatcher who receives the call will question the unit in the field about the "nature of the Signal 13," so the police can be told.
- ▶ Before sending the assistance that the Signal 13 elicits when received from law enforcement personnel in the field, the law enforcement dispatcher will require a detailed explanation of the requested signal.

When calling for help, give the exact location where you can meet rather than the location of the vehicle and the aggressor. Suggest an approach route that avoids passing the scene of the incident en route to your location. Make the law enforcement personnel responding to your assistance aware that violence has erupted. *Never send an unknowing law enforcement officer into a dangerous situation that you have already left.*

Once the dispatcher has acknowledged the call for assistance, you must supply information relating to the following:

▶ The number of aggressors involved
▶ The number and type of injuries
▶ The number and type of weapons involved
▶ The make, color, body style, and license number of the vehicle involved
▶ The direction of travel whenever the vehicle leaves the scene before the law enforcement personnel arrive

Whenever a unit in the field requests law enforcement assistance because of violence, the dispatcher should automatically send an additional EMS unit and a supervisor to the location of the unit requesting assistance. Do not send additional units to the original location of the incident, which is now the center of the danger zone.

▼   **SURVIVAL TIPS**   ▼

1 You are on the scene of an incident to help someone in need of assistance. If you lose control of the situation, you lose the ability to provide an acceptable level of service. Return to the unit, and leave the danger zone.

2 Develop a code word signifying that a weapon has been found on the patient. Make the code word something simple, for example, calling your partner by the wrong name. Plan in advance for the name you will use. All team members within hearing distance will instantly recognize the potential danger when they hear the code word.

3 In the case of armed patients, you must immobilize their hands. They may still be able to kick you, but they cannot shoot you with their feet; they may be able to bite you, but they cannot shoot you with their mouth; and they may be able to butt you, but they cannot shoot you with their head. Secure their hands and they cannot reach their weapon.

4 If you take a firearm from a patient, do not attempt to unload the weapon. All weapons are different in sensitivity: some have shaved-down trigger mechanisms, and certain semiautomatics are carried in the cocked position with the safety "on." You may not know that the safety had been moved to the off position during the accident, and the gun may discharge.

5 If the patient becomes violent in the back of the unit, do not try restraint. Stop the unit and get out. Make sure the driver takes the keys and that you have a portable radio to call for assistance. Treat this type of situation the same way you would if you were backing the unit away from a danger zone. The only difference is that the unit is now the danger zone, and you are backing away to a safe area on foot.

5

RESIDENTIAL INCIDENTS

Emergency response personnel are frequently called to residential areas to assist a person injured in an assault or domestic dispute. The experienced responder will automatically exercise caution on any call that involves injuries resulting from violent action. Calls involving violence are *not* the only ones that require caution. You should question the cause any time you receive a call reporting "severe bleeding." An "attempted suicide" could turn into a homicide, with *you* as the victim. Do not assume you will find friendly faces at the scene of a "nature unknown" call. Even an innocent "sick person" can unexpectedly become aggressive. A petite, elderly patient can suddenly become violent and powerful as a result of medication toxicity or overdose. Any call has the potential of becoming a dangerous situation (Figure 5-1).

Many times the caller is too hysterical to provide complete information. Dispatchers should share this knowledge with the responding unit. Ask yourself, Why was the caller hysterical? Until you can answer this question, proceed with caution.

Modern communications do not guarantee that the information received from dispatch is accurate and complete. In many situations the details are repeated several times before they reach the responding unit. A comparison of the amount of information provided by the caller to that received by the responding unit may resemble an inverted pyramid (Figure 5-2). Each time a call is filtered, chances are increased that information vital to the responding unit will be omitted by the person providing the data or not accurately recorded by the person on the receiving end of the call. For

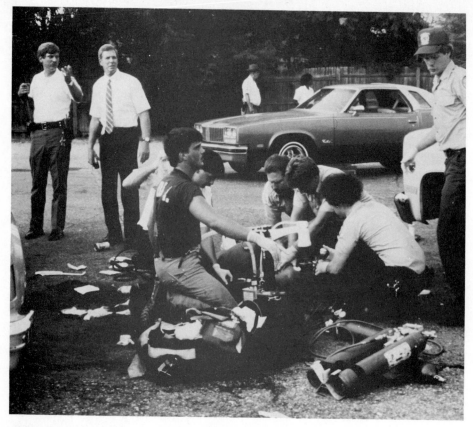

FIGURE 5-1

When the engine company and paramedic units arrived on the scene of this shooting before the police, the gunman was still on the parking lot and would not allow them to approach the victim. *(Courtesy Keith R. Hammack, Glen Burnie, Md.)*

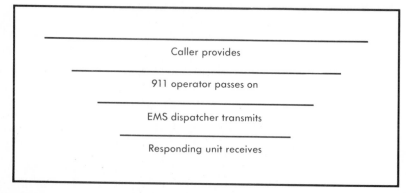

Caller provides

911 operator passes on

EMS dispatcher transmits

Responding unit receives

FIGURE 5-2

Comparison of amount of information provided by calling party with amount received by responding unit.

example, a caller to 911 reports "a person having a heart attack in a blue van on the parking lot of Albertson's Market." The 911 operator relays to the EMS dispatcher, "heart attack in a van on the parking lot of Albertson's Market." The EMS dispatcher sends an Advanced Life Support (ALS) unit to "a heart attack in the parking lot of Albertson's Market." The ALS crew members record and respond to "a heart attack at Albertson's Market." On arrival, they see more than 50 vehicles of all descriptions in the parking lot and look inside the store for the stricken person.

Responders must never assume that they have received enough information to disregard the potential for danger on any call. Before entering a residence, use a systematic approach to increase your chances of avoiding potentially dangerous situations. The technique of approach that you develop and perfect may not be required on every call, but if your systematic approach is practiced and refined on every response, you will be prepared when a dangerous situation occurs.

AN ESCALATING INCIDENT

The following incident is an example of what can happen to you when least expected. While you read the narrative, which was provided by one of the firefighters involved, consider your reactions if you had been in this situation:

At approximately 6 PM on 8 September 1982, the crew from Engine 46 was sitting in the kitchen of its quarters with a visiting police officer. Conversation stopped when the officer's portable radio broke squelch and began to broadcast the details of the arrest of a dope dealer occurring less than 3 blocks from the station.

Resisting arrest, the dealer ran down the street with two police officers in foot pursuit. The police fired shots, and the suspect dived through a glass storm door at a residence located in a group of row houses on Belvedere Avenue. Although the dealer had a massive laceration on his upper leg, he was still able to break free from the grasp of the officer who had reached through the broken door and grabbed him. This officer sustained a laceration on the arm and had to stop the pursuit. Four officers were needed to subdue the fighting suspect and remove him from the basement of the house.

Medic 14 was dispatched to "assist an injured police officer in a residence, Belvedere Avenue." On arrival, the medic unit was surprised to see four police officers struggling to control a profusely bleeding male. (The injured officer had gone to the hospital before the medic unit arrived.) Before the crew could reach the patient, he collapsed at the front door in full cardiac arrest. By this time a substantial crowd had gathered. The people assumed that the man had been beaten into submission by the police, and they started to turn ugly. While assisting the cardiac patient, the medic unit called for an engine company backup.

Engine 46 was dispatched to "assist Medic 14 with a cardiac patient in a residence, Belvedere Avenue." The engine company had to work its way through an estimated crowd of 200 angry neighbors to reach the patient. After being stabilized, the patient was transported to the nearest hospital where he later died. Following their procedure for this type of incident, the police stopped all routine patrol within a 6-square-block area surrounding the house on Belvedere Avenue. This action further upset the neighborhood residents.

A street box was received in the same immediate area at about 8 PM—it was a false alarm. An "unknown type fire" call was received from the same location at about 8:30 PM—it was a trash fire. Both times the engine company encountered large crowds but was able to return to quarters without confrontation.

Shortly after 9 PM, Engine 46 was dispatched to a "Medic standby, unknown type of injured person" at the same residence on Belvedere Avenue. The street appeared quiet, but two patrol cars and four police officers were assigned to escort the engine to the location. At the residence a group of eight adult males awaited the arriving crew. The fire lieutenant, both firefighters, and all four police officers entered the residence to assess the reported patient. Finding no visible injuries, the fire and police personnel exited to the front porch where two persons from an arriving medic unit met them. While they conferred on the patient's condition, an unknown assailant began shooting at them. Bullets struck tree limbs 3 feet over their heads. Everyone dived for cover and scrambled into the house. The police radioed that they were under fire. Even though the shooting continued, the residents of the house ordered all fire and police personnel to leave.

The pump operator on Engine 46 had remained with the engine and observed three people who were acting suspiciously enter the house across the street just before the shooting. The operator backed the engine down the street and was turning the engine around when the shots rang out. He notified dispatch that there was trouble at the scene. The battalion chief, not knowing that the lieutenant and two firefighters were not on board, ordered the engine to return to quarters immediately.

A police helicopter and a squad of police officers made a sweep down Belvedere Avenue so the crew could exit the house. But since the engine had left the scene, the crew was stranded. They hid behind a group of cars on the parking lot of a nearby supermarket. The sounds of gunshots, breaking glass, and yelling were all around them when the lieutenant radioed for help. After about 20 minutes a patrol car found and returned the crew to the engine house safely.[1]

Fortunately, these kinds of situations are rare. However, if you were involved in a similar incident before you finished reading this book, would you be prepared?

ARRIVING ON THE SCENE

Emergency service units habitually arrive on the scene with flashing lights and wailing sirens. Personnel jump from the unit, fill both arms with equipment, run the length of the sidewalk, and charge through the door with very little thought for their own safety. This approach has no element of surprise; it is more of a "Here we are, where's the patient?" type of arrival. For your own safety, turn off the siren and warning lights far enough in advance to prevent the occupants of the residence from hearing and seeing your arrival (Figure 5-3). If the address is located in a subdivision, warning lights and sirens can usually be turned off when entering the neighborhood. If the call is on a through street, turn them off a couple of

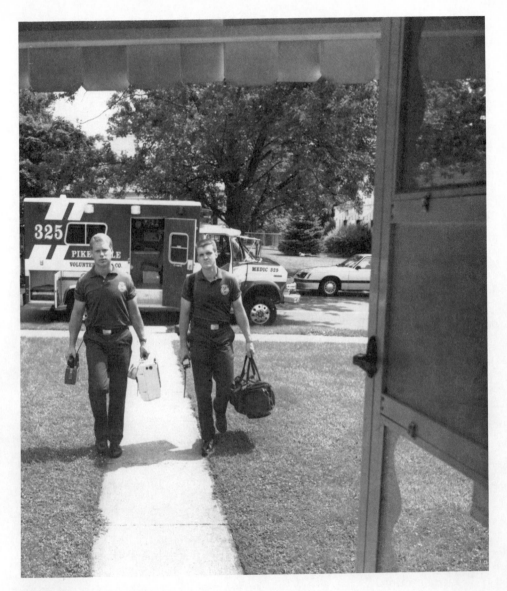

FIGURE 5-3
Properly prepared paramedics do not charge into the unknown. They first consider their own safety and then that of the patient.

blocks before the address. Traffic conditions are usually less congested in the early morning and late at night than during normal business hours and early evening, so use the siren only when traffic conditions dictate. Be aware that at night a siren can be heard from a great distance. Unnecessary use of the sirens and emergency warning lights will have three results.

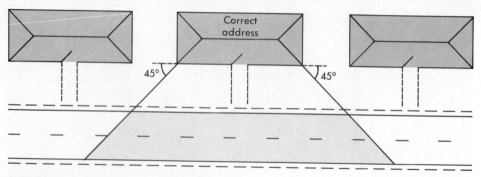

FIGURE 5-4

To prevent the occupants in the house from observing your arrival, do not stop
your unit in the shaded area.

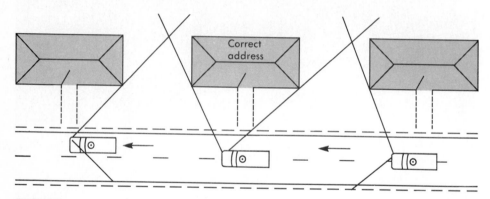

FIGURE 5-5

Positioning the unit on far side of the residence permits a three-sided observation.

> ▶ It will eliminate the element of surprise.
> ▶ It will damage public relations on the legitimate call. Many people
>   are embarrassed to use our services. They appreciate units showing
>   discretion.
> ▶ It will draw a crowd when you arrive on the scene. In many areas,
>   having a crowd converge around the unit is not safe.

If you stop the unit directly in front of the structure, the occupants
can watch your every move and still remain unseen. Stop the unit approximately one hundred feet from the residence. A rule of thumb is to stop before reaching an imaginary line that runs 45 degrees from the corner of the
residence or continue past an imaginary line of the same angle on the opposite corner of the residence (Figure 5-4). Pulling past the residence is op-
timal because you can observe three sides of the structure before you leave
the unit (Figure 5-5). As you approach the residence, you see the near side;

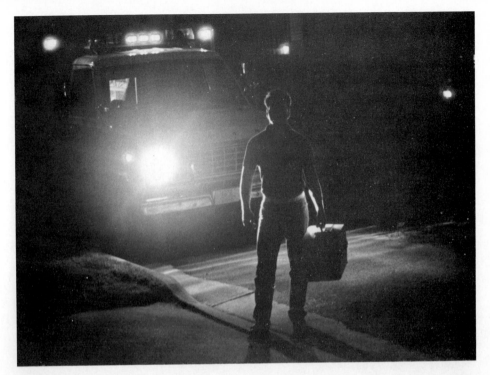

FIGURE 5-6
Night arrivals dictate that headlights be turned off before exiting the unit to avoid
backlighting the rescuer. If it is necessary to park the unit on a public street,
parking lights and/or emergency flashers should be turned on to alert passing
motorists.

as you slowly pass, you see the front; and after you stop the unit, you observe the far side. You need to learn as much as possible about the situation outside and inside the residence while maintaining your element of
surprise (Figure 5-6).

Enter long driveways with caution. Position your unit where you probably cannot be seen from the residence but close enough to move the necessary equipment efficiently to the door (Figure 5-7). If no cover is available, position your unit near enough to the residence to provide the required service. If the driveway configuration permits, position the unit in
line with the corner of the residence. Finally, turn the unit around to ensure
a direct route of exit from the property. Escaping forward is much easier
than backward. If the response is after dark and enough natural light is
present, turn the headlights off before entering the driveway. If necessary,
use the parking lights to make the approach.

Garden apartment and townhouse complexes present unique approach
problems because of overcrowded parking lots and many dead-end streets

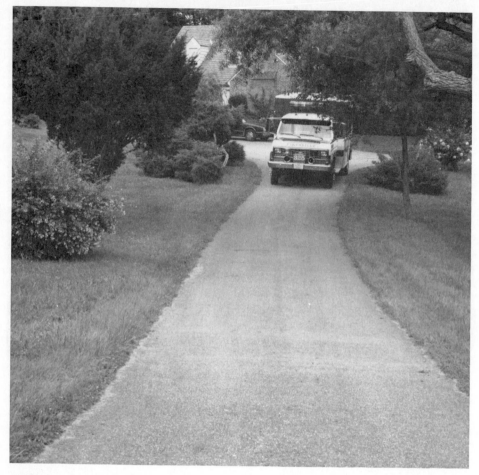

FIGURE 5-7
A properly positioned medic unit at the end of a long driveway commands a view
of two sides of the residence while not being in direct line with any windows or
doors.

and cul-de-sacs. When approaching a multistory apartment building, scan
upper-floor windows, patios, and the roof line for signs of a setup. After
you complete the scan, do not look straight up; a falling object may strike
you in the face. Wear helmet protection whenever you are working near a
multistory building.

Many apartment buildings have security doors at the main entrance.
People gain entry to the building by sounding the doorbell of the apartment
they want to enter, and the occupant unlocks the main entrance door (Figure 5-8). To gain access to this type of building and maintain the element of
surprise, ring any doorbell *except* the correct one. Use caution on every
alarm involving high-density occupancies.

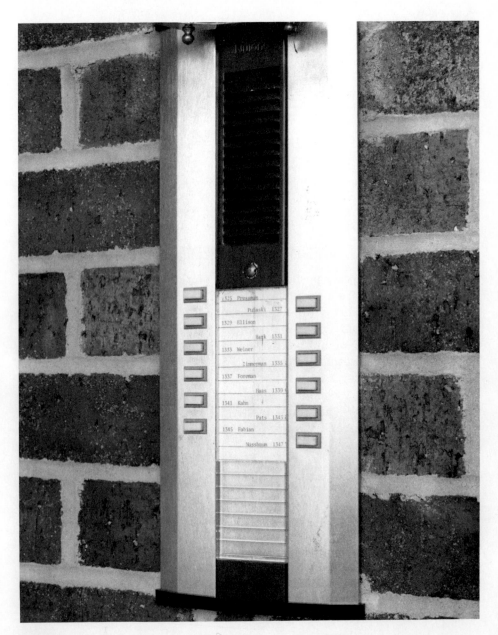

FIGURE 5-8
Doorbell pushbuttons on the front entrance of an apartment building with a security door.

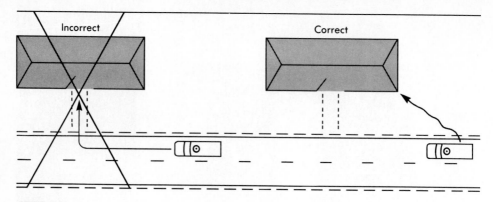

FIGURE 5-9
Approaching the residence from an angle permits the rescuers to maintain the element of surprise.

APPROACHING THE RESIDENCE

When you properly position the unit, you will be in a position to approach a residence from an angle. This will keep you out of the normal line of sight. The occupant will be looking for you to approach from a frontal position and not from across the lawn at an angle (Figure 5-9).

Two personnel should be used for residential approaches so that each crew member can watch for the other's safety. In addition, the amount of equipment needed for a residential response is usually more than one person can carry. When removing equipment from the unit, do not slam the compartment doors—shut them quietly.

While you approach the residence, devote your total concentration to the area surrounding the structure (Figure 5-10). This is not the time for idle conversation. Use all of your senses to gather information about the incident:

- ▶ What do you see when you look through the windows? (Do not stand directly in front of the window. Stand to the side and several steps away from the wall.)
- ▶ What do you hear from the inside?
- ▶ Do you see or hear a struggle?
- ▶ Do you see any high-threat weapons?
- ▶ Do you hear loud or abusive voices?
- ▶ How many voices are there?
- ▶ Do you feel that the environment is safe for you to enter?

After you reach the front entrance, analyze all the information obtained during the approach before announcing your presence and entering the residence. Do not knock on the door until you are ready to go inside. If you doubt the urgency of the need for medical assistance, perform a primary survey from the front porch *before* making your presence known. If

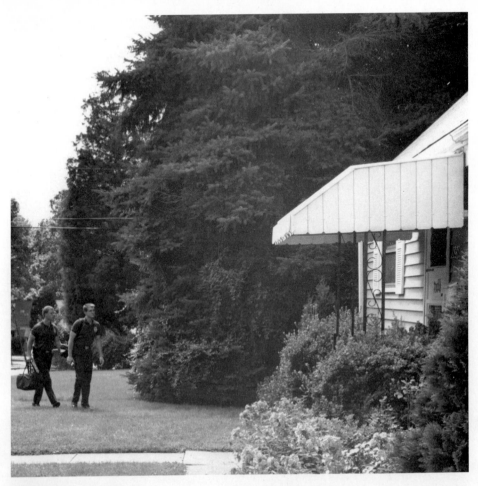

FIGURE 5-10
When you near the residence, shift your concentration to the structure.

the occupants are yelling at one another, they are conscious and their airways are patent. If they continue to argue, it is doubtful that either is bleeding profusely, and their need for medical assistance is probably not urgent.

Anytime danger is indicated, abort the approach and back away to the unit. Do not turn your back to the residence—keep the source of your apprehension in sight. Remember, withdrawing to an area of safety is not the same as leaving the scene. Until you have determined that no medical assistance is required, do not leave the scene.

After you are back in the unit, call for law enforcement assistance and move the unit away from the building to an area of relative safety. Inform the dispatcher of the problem and where you will meet the police officers, possibly at the nearest intersection. When they arrive at the scene, brief the officers on the situation before they approach the residence.

▼   SURVIVAL TIPS   ▼

1   Before starting the approach, remove all loose items (such as change and keys) from your pockets. You do not want to carry anything unnecessary that may destroy your element of surprise.

2   While in the unit, keep the unit radio's volume level just loud enough for clear communications. Start each response and approach with the volume on portable radios turned very low. Increase the volume only when needed.

3   Determine if the attempted suicide is a *medical suicide* or a *traumatic suicide* before arriving on the scene. A person who has swallowed a bottle of pills is usually not going to hurt you; however, the person who had an unsuccessful suicide attempt using a weapon may turn that weapon on you.

4   On a reported shooting, stabbing, or traumatic suicide, consider stopping the unit a block or more before the address. Remain with the unit until law enforcement personnel have arrived on the scene and declared the area safe.

5   A person who has requested assistance from the emergency services does not have a "signed contract." If you feel your personal safety is endangered, you are under no obligation to enter the residence.

6

ENTERING A STRUCTURE

Consider the following situation: Paramedics responding to a reported suicide were standing at the front door of the residence when they heard a scream from inside. The door opened and a man holding a knife in his outstretched hand came running out of the house. If they had not jumped to the side as he passed, one of the paramedics would probably have been impaled on the knife.

A door does not need to be open to expose a rescuer to a hazardous situation. Weapons have been fired through closed doors to try to injure whoever was standing on the other side (Figure 6-1).[1] Seasoned veterans teach new personnel to avoid positioning themselves in front of any door, closed or open, until they have completed all safety checks and the response team is ready to enter the structure.

POSITIONING AT THE DOOR

The front door to most homes opens inward. When approaching a door, stand to the doorknob side of the entrance to announce your presence (Figure 6-2). The occupant should open the door far enough to look around the jamb and see you. If you are standing on the hinged side of the door, the occupant can observe you by opening the door slightly. However, you would have a limited view of conditions inside the room and would not be certain of your safety (Figure 6-3). Always stand in a line with the door frame rather than with the Sheetrock wall. Door frames are usually constructed from wood or metal and offer better protection than Sheetrock

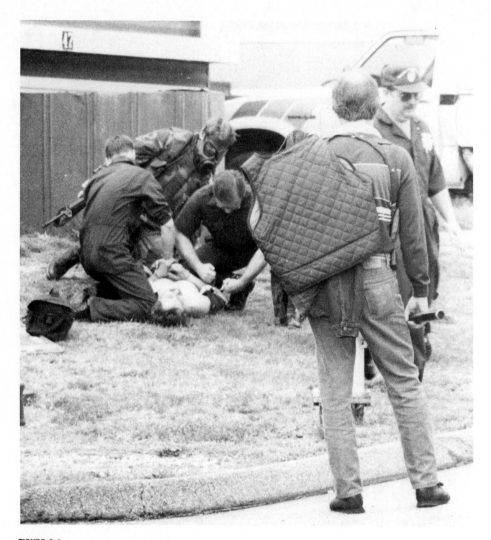

FIGURE 6-1

Paramedics and SWAT personnel care for a man who had fired an arrow through a closed door at approaching paramedics. *(Courtesy Allen Hafner, Howard County Police Department, Ellicott City, Md.)*

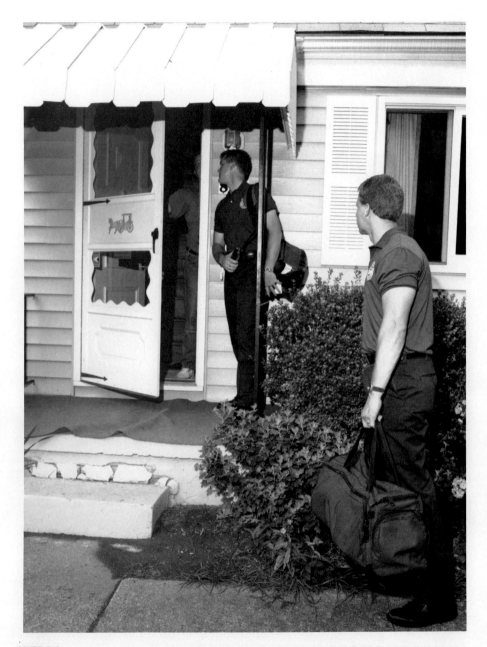

FIGURE 6-2
Stand on the doorknob side of the entrance when announcing your arrival.

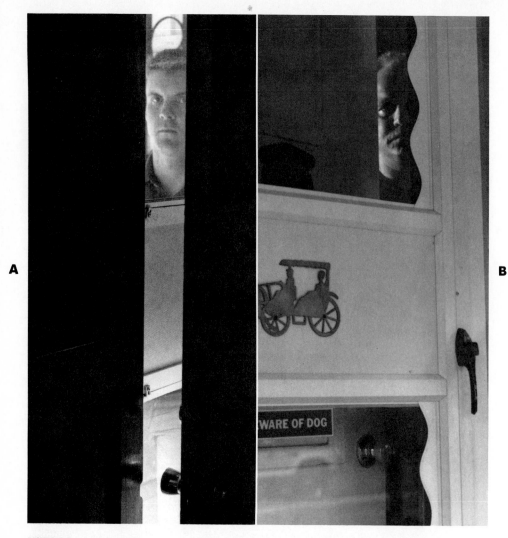

FIGURE 6-3
A, When rescuers stand on the hinged side of the door, **B,** the occupants can observe the rescuer without exposing themselves.

when a bullet is fired through the wall. If the entryway includes an outer door (a screen or storm door), remain on the doorknob side of the door that opens inward (Figure 6-4).

When responding to garden apartments or high-rise apartment buildings, you may not be able to stand to the side of the door because of the construction features of the building. One option is to knock on the door and quickly move several steps down the stairway before announcing yourself (Figure 6-5). Before returning to the front of the door, wait until the occupant opens the door and acts appropriately.

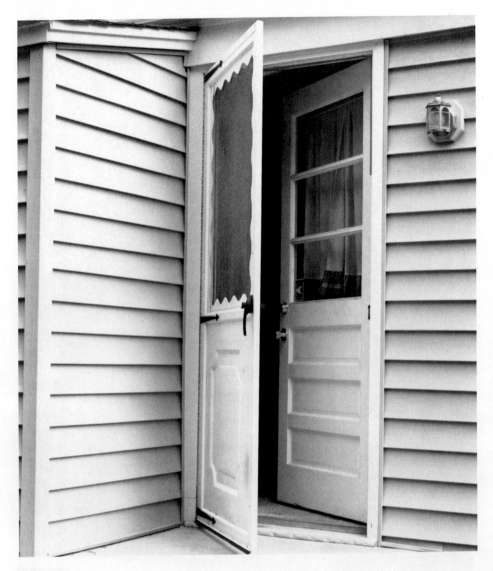

FIGURE 6-4
Some outer doors are hinged on the opposite side of the door frame as the primary door. Remain on the doorknob side of the primary door when establishing initial contact with the occupants.

When using an elevator in high-rises, set it on manual or fireman's service (Figure 6-6). Silence the alarm before ascending, and hold the car on the floor of the medical emergency (with the door open) until all members of the team are ready to descend. Locate any stairwells before using the elevator. Visualize their location in relation to the elevator. You may need to use the stairs as a second means of escape. When you reach the proper floor, check

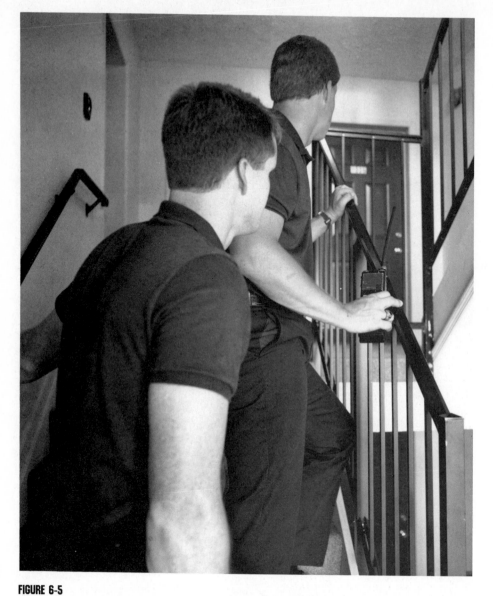

FIGURE 6-5
When construction features prevent standing to the side of the entrance, quickly
move down the stairs after knocking on the door.

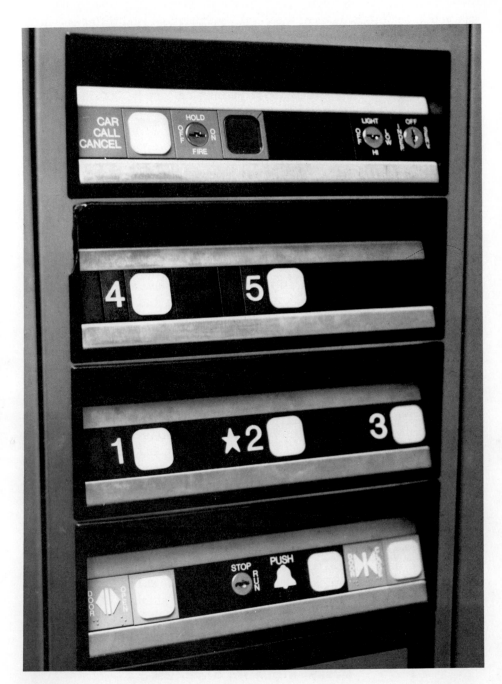

FIGURE 6-6
Typical elevator control panel.

the stairwell doors and make sure they are unlocked and free to open before you knock on the door of the apartment that reported the emergency.

If the entrance door to the residence is open on your arrival, do *not* go
inside without permission; knock and wait to be admitted because of the
following reasons:

> ▸ Entering a residence without permission can be considered tres-
>   passing or breaking and entering.
> ▸ You may be in the wrong location.[2]
> ▸ It may be a setup. If intentionally lured into a violent environment,
>   you may be seriously injured or killed.[3]

When you knock on the door and announce, "Paramedics," "Fire department," or "Rescue squad," wait for someone to come to the door before
moving in front of the opening. If someone calls "come in" without coming
to the door, be wary. Ask them if they can step outside to talk with you before you enter. If they say they cannot, find out why. Try to get the occupant to move into your line of sight. If they refuse without a good reason,
consider withdrawing to the unit and requesting law enforcement assistance. When the injured person claims to be alone and unable to come to
the door, proceed with caution.

MOVING THROUGH THE ENTRANCE WAY

When your team decides to enter the residence, move without hesita-
tion. Do not pause in the opening. Law enforcement personnel refer to the
opening to any room as the *kill zone* (Figure 6-7). The occupants can watch
the entrance without moving, but you have to turn your head to see the entire room. The time it takes you to locate and recognize a dangerous situation from the entryway may not be enough to save you from a fatal injury.

The first rescuer to enter the residence should look between the door
frame and the hinge side of the door while opening the door as far as possible. If it does not open fully, someone may be behind the door. When in
doubt, do not enter the room.

Usually, the last member of the rescue team entering the residence
closes the door out of respect for the occupant. Leave the door ajar whenever the exact location of the incident was not clear at the time of the call.
If the original rescue team questions the continued stability of the incident,
the crew should leave the door partially open so that other emergency response teams can hear inside the residence before entering (Figure 6-8).

MOVING WITHIN THE STRUCTURE

Ask the occupant to show you the location of the patient. Let the occupant lead you through the residence. You will have the quickest route to the
victim and be protected from an unexpected attack. The occupant unknow-

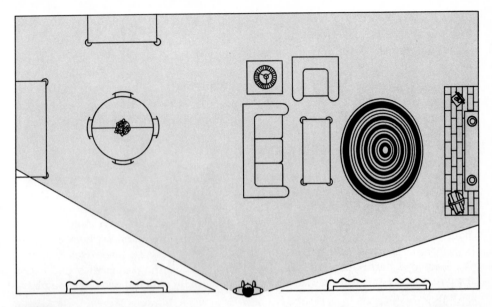

FIGURE 6-7
Standing in the kill zone.

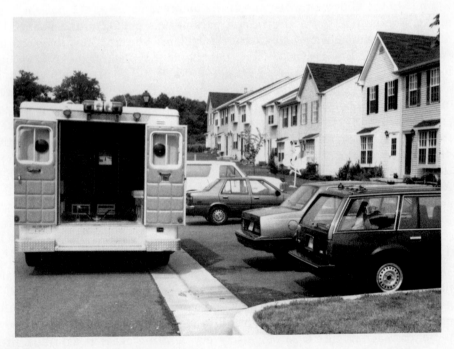

FIGURE 6-8
First unit on the scene probably met someone waiting to identify the correct residence. Following units may not have this assistance.

ingly acts as a shield for team members and provides a few extra moments to react if the situation deteriorates.

The person who answers the door is usually a family member or close friend of the patient and will reduce the anxiety level of the patient by leading the rescue team into the room. The victim is already nervous because of the emergency and will feel reassured if a familiar face comes into the room before several strangers with their arms full of ominous-looking equipment. The advantage of following the occupant to the patient is illustrated in the following example:

A woman calls for an ambulance because her husband is having difficulty breathing. She meets the paramedics at the front door with a worried look on her face, points to the stairs, and says, "He's in the bedroom." The paramedics run up the stairs, hurry into the bedroom without knocking, and slide to a stop when the man rolls out of bed with a 9 mm semiautomatic pistol pointed at them. His wife had not told him she was calling the fire department. All he knew was that two strangers had burst unannounced into his bedroom. If the paramedics had asked the wife to take them to the bedroom, this potentially violent encounter may have been prevented.

If the victim has a trauma injury, do not let other occupants in the residence out of your sight until you determine who or what caused the injury. In one incident, paramedics were treating a man with multiple stab wounds to the abdomen when one of the paramedics asked the patient who did it. The patient pointed over the paramedic's shoulder and said, "She did." The paramedics turned to see the woman who had met them at the front door standing between them and the door with a large knife in her hand.[4]

If one of the occupants in the room with the patient starts to leave (no matter what reason they give), have a member of the rescue team accompany them. If no extra emergency services personnel are available, say that you need assistance and ask the person to hold the IV bag, steady the patient's legs, or perform some other small task that will keep the person in the room and within your line of sight. This action will reduce the possibility of an unidentified antagonist obtaining a weapon and returning to the scene.

WEAPONS IN THE RESIDENCE

While proceeding to the patient's location, scan the rooms you are passing through for weapons. Make a mental note of the location of both high-threat and low-threat weapons (see Chapter 3). After reaching the proper room, pay particular attention to weapons that may be within the patient's reach (Figure 6-9). Move scissors, knitting needles, ashtrays, fireplace pokers, and other dangerous articles out of the patient's reach to make room for your equipment. Whenever possible, place sharp objects under furniture or between cushions. Avoid touching or moving high-threat

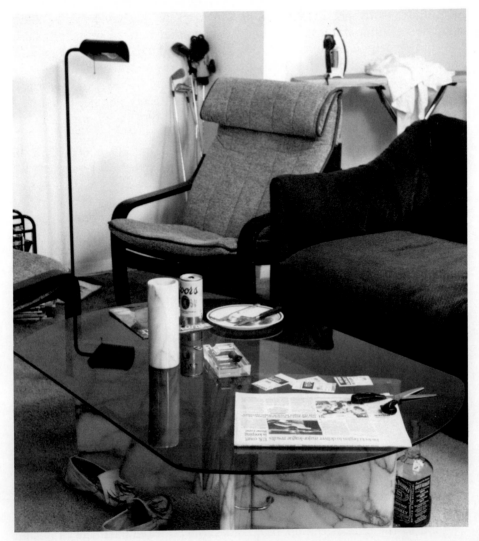

FIGURE 6-9
Identify the possible threats to your safety in this scene.

weapons such as guns and knives; the weapon may have been used in a crime, and if you pick it up, you may destroy irreplaceable evidence. When you encounter a gun or a knife, move the patient away from the weapon rather than the weapon away from the patient. Use an excuse, such as lack of light or room, for your action.

More potential weapons are found in a kitchen than in any other room in a residence. These weapons are within easy reach from any part of most kitchens. When forced to provide patient care in a kitchen, be extremely alert to the possibilities for injury.

Today, many people have loaded firearms in the house for personal protection. A nightstand next to the bed, a dresser drawer, or an end table next to a favorite chair in the family room are popular locations to conceal these weapons. You may not see a weapon but, for your own safety, assume it is there. Many people that own weapons have no training in the proper use of firearms. The weapon may be poorly constructed or need repair. A round may be in the chamber, and the safety, if it has one, is probably off. For your own safety, avoid picking up a strange gun.

Do not pick up a weapon and put it in the jump kit or drug box for safekeeping. The weapon is not your property, and you do not have the authority to remove it from a residence. If you put the weapon in your equipment, you can be charged with stealing, no matter how innocent the action or how sincere your intentions. If you must move a weapon, make a mental note of its original location. Give this information to the police officer writing the report and include the site on your incident report. Always inform law enforcement personnel of the location of all firearms you have found in the residence.

Being aware of the potential presence of firearms within the residence should prepare the emergency service responder to make timely and effective decisions regarding patient treatment.

▼   SURVIVAL TIPS   ▼

1 When the person who opens the door is belligerent, you are not obligated to enter. Do not try to gain entry when you are met with hostility.

2 Always move *down* the stairs to await the opening of a door. If you move up the stairs, your avenue of escape will be cut off if violence erupts.

3 Attempt a window entry to a residence only after all conventional methods have failed. The occupant may mistake you as a threat and take aggressive action against you. If you decide to enter this way, always stand to the side of the opening and shout, "Fire department," "Rescue squad," or "Paramedics," several times before entering the window.[5]

4 Do not allow a person who has been involved in a dispute with the victim to assist with patient care; this may precipitate further violence. Use caution when selecting occupants for assistance in packaging the patient.

5 Whenever possible, avoid treating a patient that is within reach of any weapon. Either move the weapon or move the patient.

7

DOMESTIC ENCOUNTERS

On the evening of 29 May 1987, a man in New Lancaster Valley, Pennsylvania, reported that he had been assaulted by his son during a domestic dispute and requested the police. Shortly afterward, a structure fire was reported at the same location. As the responding police and fire personnel approached the house, shots were fired at them from inside. Before reaching safety, one firefighter was killed and another firefighter and a state trooper were wounded.[1] The wounded firefighter died 4 days later.[2] Although the situation appeared calm when emergency services personnel arrived, it escalated into a deadly dispute in a matter of seconds. Unexpected violence may erupt during your next response to a domestic dispute.

Domestic disturbances are considered to be one of the most dangerous situations law enforcement officers encounter. Emergency services personnel must be aware of the danger involved with these incidents and handle them with extreme caution.

If a violent or physical dispute is in progress at a residence when you arrive, wait for law enforcement assistance before you enter. Sometimes tempers subside when the rescue team arrives on the scene and flare up again after you start patient care. When this happens, separate the fighting parties as quickly as possible, but do not stand between them (Figure 7-1). Use voice commands, eye contact, and body language to manipulate the people to turn away from each other until they are back to back. After the individuals involved in the dispute lose sight of one another, the level of tension is reduced.

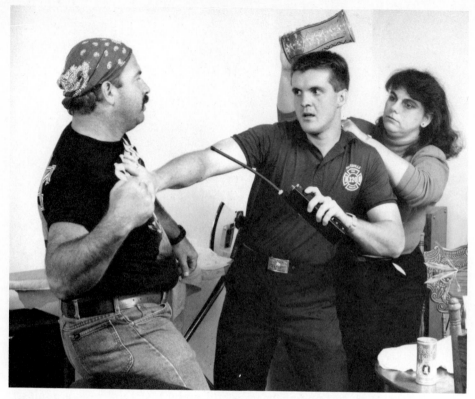

FIGURE 7-1
Do not stand between fighting parties. You may be the one who receives the most injuries.

CALM THE SITUATION WITH VOICE CONTROL

Your voice is the most effective tool you can use to keep out of trouble in a dispute. Your speed, tone, and vocabulary will affect the outcome of every situation.

Control the tone of your voice. Do not sound overly authoritative but at the same time avoid sounding weak. Analyze each situation before you decide what tone to use. If your voice conveys to the participants in the dispute that they control the situation, you are in trouble.

Be careful in choosing your words; certain words may further antagonize the person you are trying to calm. Do not use condescending words such as *sport, buddy,* or *pal.* Avoid the terms *gramps* and *pop* when speaking with older people. Individuals involved in domestic situations are already irrational, and using the wrong word may cause aggression to be directed toward you. Remember, everybody has a button—a sensitive area that causes anger. If your button is pushed, back off and try to remain calm. Losing control may result in your demeaning the patient or anyone associated with the incident. Never retaliate by pushing tempers out of control.

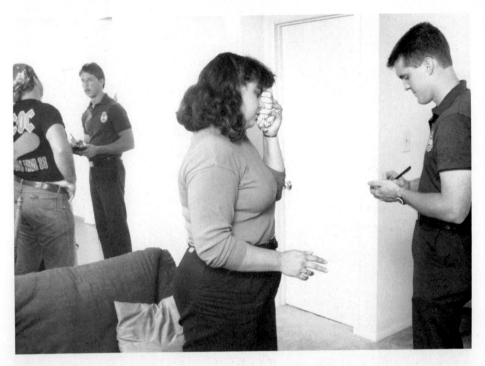

FIGURE 7-2
If you maintain eye contact and conversation with the individual as you begin to move, the participant will likely move wherever you lead.

Know your temper level and your likely reaction when someone antagonizes you. Know your partner's weak points; you will be better prepared if your partner loses control.

Talk to people with the same respect that you expect from them. Regardless of your personal opinion of the person you are treating, address the patient as "Sir" or "Ma'am." Ask, "What's your name?" Introduce yourself, and stay on that level throughout the encounter.

Never forget that you are a professional. Your duty is to act in a professional manner, no matter how unpleasant the situation may be. This begins when you knock on the front door. When the occupants ask who you are, tell them and then ask for permission to enter the residence. Wait until you receive permission before you open the door, and then wipe your feet before going inside. Once inside, separate and keep the occupants individually engaged in conversation. These little things make the difference between a successful and an unsuccessful situation.

TURN THE INDIVIDUAL WITH EYE CONTACT

Speak and establish eye contact with one of the individuals involved in the dispute. After eye contact is made, continue talking to this individual and slowly move in a circular direction away from the other person (Figure

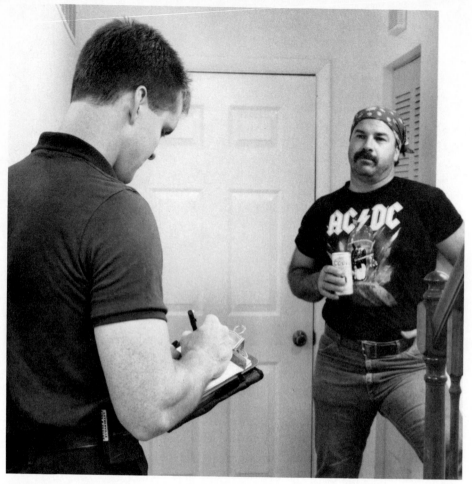

FIGURE 7-3
Do not allow any of the participants in the dispute to position themselves between you and the door.

7-2). Your partner should be doing the same thing with the other person but moving in the opposite direction. Showing concern and sympathy aids in gaining that person's attention and confidence. Do not grab and turn the person; a discreet movement of your eyes and body will give the desired effect.

When you execute this movement, do not place yourself in a tactically unsound position. One common mistake is to spin the person into a position between the rescuer and the primary or secondary means of egress (Figure 7-3).

Do not loose sight of your partner during this move. Use your peripheral vision to watch all other activity in the area, (Figure 7-4) while con-

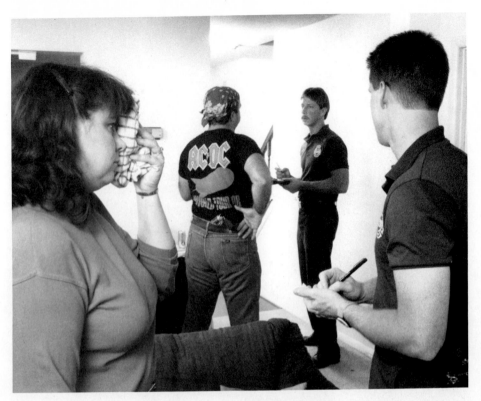

FIGURE 7-4
Using your peripheral vision, look for weapons on the individual your partner is interviewing.

tinuing a conversation with your own antagonist. If you see a weapon in the waistband or back pocket of the other person's trousers, warn your partner by using a prearranged code word, such as calling your partner by the wrong name.

BODY LANGUAGE

The way you stand when talking to the disputing parties influences the situation. If you enter a room and assume an aggressive posture (such as with feet apart and hands on your hips), you are inviting abuse. Standing with your arms crossed over your chest may also bring a challenge from one of the involved parties. This gesture conveys the message, "My mind is made up; I cannot be swayed." An *interview stance* should be nonthreatening and provide a high degree of safety to the rescuer (Figure 7-5). Defending against aggressive movements toward you is discussed in Chapter 13.

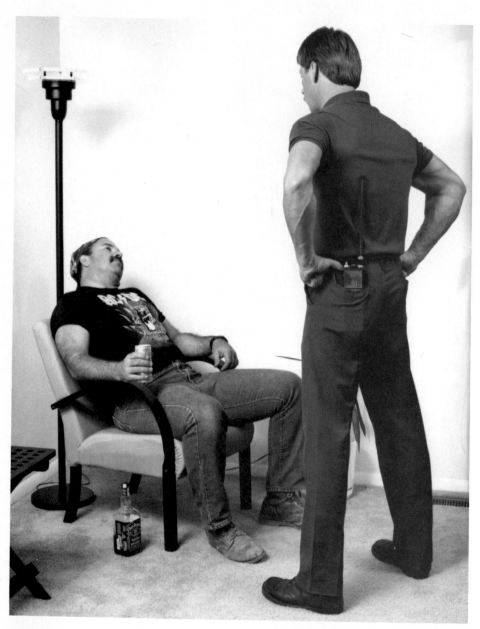

FIGURE 7-5
Do not stand in a threatening or indifferent position.

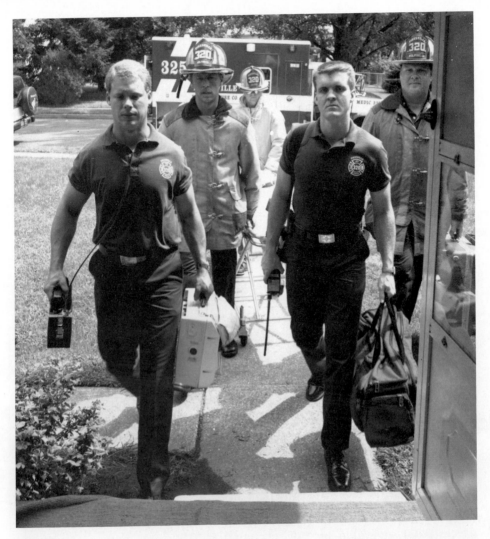

FIGURE 7-6
Using a tier system of entry prevents the occupants from feeling they are being invaded.

TIER SYSTEM OF ENTRY INTO AN UNSTABLE AREA

All units responding to an emergency rarely arrive at the same time. In most incidents, several minutes pass between the arrival of units because of unequal travel distances and delays associated with interagency notification.

Even if several units arrive on the scene at the same time, use the tier system of entry (Figure 7-6). The occupants can then adjust to your presence. If everyone charges through the door at the same time, the residents may feel overwhelmed.

The first crew to enter the building should tell the people involved in the dispute that additional personnel will be arriving on the scene to bring additional equipment or provide extra assistance. Explain to the people that you and your partner are the only ones they will be dealing with; all other personnel will remain outside or out of the way unless they are needed to assist in treatment.

If you are on the second arriving unit, knock on the door and wait for permission to enter. If the first unit has managed to settle the domestic argument and separate the parties and you unexpectedly walk through the door, the argument may start all over again. This time the anger may be aimed at you, eliciting a "WHO THE HELL ARE YOU?" Now you have to start at the beginning and calm the people at the scene, explain your presence, and separate the fighting parties.

USE OF BARRIERS TO SEPARATE INDIVIDUALS

Physical obstacles such as coffee tables and sofas are a psychological barrier to the fighting parties. Although it is easy to jump over or walk around most furniture, these objects can serve as a barrier that will successfully separate the antagonists (Figure 7-7). Features of construction such as curtain walls, room dividers, and breakfast bars can also separate people. They may block the line of sight between the fighting parties, which automatically calms the situation. If you cannot see the person you are fighting, it is difficult to continue the fight. When these barriers are used, position yourself where you can see your partner (Figure 7-8).

DISTRACTION TECHNIQUES

Sometimes a domestic dispute will flare up after the parties have been successfully separated by the rescue team. Often one person thinks the other person is telling the rescuer something that is not true or requesting the rescuer to pass a message to the police about the other person. If the party that you are treating or interviewing suddenly turns away from you and starts yelling at the other party, quickly employ a distraction technique to break the person's train of thought. Do this as soon as possible to prevent the argument from escalating to its original level. Tell the person your pen ran out of ink and ask for another one so you can write down some necessary information. Ask to see a driver's license or an insurance card for billing. When you start talking about sending a bill for your services, you will usually get the person's undivided attention. Ask unnecessary questions that require more than a "yes" or "no" answer. Always write down the answers—this will buy you time while your partner works with the other person involved in the dispute.

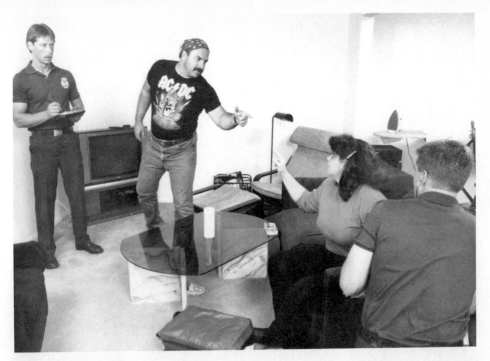

FIGURE 7-7

Furniture is a barrier between the parties.

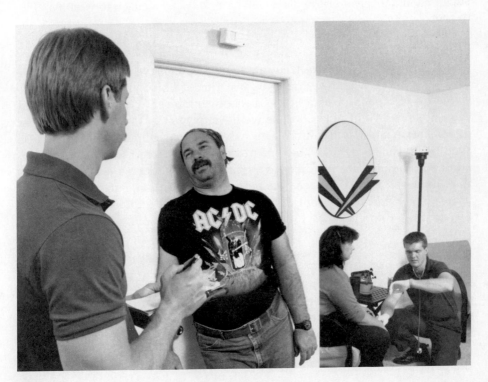

FIGURE 7-8

Never lose sight of your partner when separating fighting parties.

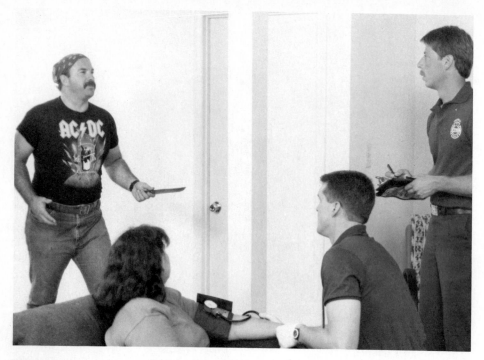

FIGURE 7-9
Do not permit anyone to leave the room alone; the person may return with a
weapon.

If the person you are treating attempts to leave the room, continue
with the interview and say that you are almost finished. The claim, "I only
want to get a pack of cigarettes," can be countered with, "We prefer that
you not smoke right now because we have oxygen in the room." If the person insists, follow and continue to ask questions about the incident. Depending on the severity of the disagreement, the person may be going after
a weapon to continue the dispute (Figure 7-9). Your presence may discour-
age this possibility. If you see the person get a weapon, run back and warn
your partner and the patient that the situation may explode. *Leave the residence immediately!*

AVOIDING THE VIOLENT SITUATION

If the person adamantly refuses to allow you to follow, do not insist to
the point that causes violence to erupt. Permit the person to leave and remain with your partner and the patient. As soon as the person is out of
sight, you and your partner should leave the residence. If possible, take the
patient with you, even if you have to use an unorthodox means of moving
the patient. If the patient hesitates or starts to argue, leave the patient be-

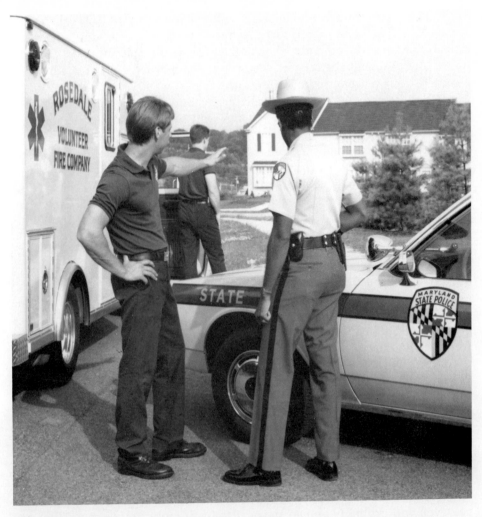

FIGURE 7-10
Do not send the local police to the house without first informing them of the
nature of the call.

hind. Do not gather your equipment; exit the residence and call for law enforcement assistance from a safe location.

Tell the dispatcher where to have the police meet your unit (possibly
at the nearest intersection) so that you can explain the situation. Do not allow the police officers to proceed to the residence without first attempting
to apprise them of the conditions inside (Figure 7-10). They were probably
given the call, "assist EMS on a domestic," and do not know that you have already been in the residence. Explain to the officers what happened when you
knocked on the door, what was said inside, what you saw, how many peo-

ple were present, and what caused you to leave the house and call for assistance. If you were unable to bring the patient out with you, advise the officers that a patient requiring emergency medical treatment is still in the house. Request that the officers secure the residence so that you can safely return to your patient and continue care.

The officers will probably call for backup before proceeding. When this happens, remain where you are and wait for additional police units to arrive. Do not approach or reenter the building until law enforcement personnel have secured the scene and declared the residence safe.

The reasons for backing away from a motor vehicle incident are discussed in Chapter 4. The same criteria apply to backing away from a hostile situation in a building. It should be difficult to convict you of abandoning your patient if you document on your report that you did the following:

▶ Feared for your personal safety because civilian personnel on the scene were uncooperative and refused to follow your instructions.
▶ Acted in self-defense.
▶ Did not take the time to gather up your equipment before leaving the hostile area.
▶ Left the hostile area at the same time as all other emergency service personnel.
▶ Did not leave the scene, only the hostile area.
▶ Called for law enforcement assistance. (Attach a copy of the police report to your report; if not available, include the police case number in your report.)
▶ Returned to the patient and continued treatment as soon as the area was declared safe by on-scene law enforcement personnel.

When either partner feels that it is time to leave a potentially hostile area, both partners must leave at the same time. At some time in your career, you will probably appear in court to testify why you believed that you were in imminent danger if you had remained in the area. You will need to explain in great detail the explosive nature of the situation and emphasize how you feared for your personal safety. When the defense attorney asks, "What did your partner do?" and you have to reply, "My partner stayed in the house," you have a serious problem. Consider how you would respond to the defense attorney's next question: "Why was it too dangerous for you to continue to treat my client, but your partner was able to stay and continue to treat the ex-spouse?" Remember, if it's bad enough for one to leave, it's bad enough for all to leave.

▼   **SURVIVAL TIPS**   ▼

1 Settling domestic disputes is not your responsibility. Your job is to provide prehospital emergency care. If care is not needed, return to service.
2 Most emergency service workers are not trained as marriage counselors, psychologists, psychiatrists, priests, or preachers. Crisis intervention is not part of your job description.
3 Never let anyone stand between you and your primary escape route.
4 Do not back yourself into a corner.
5 Plan your route of escape before you need it.
6 If violence has occurred in the residence, law enforcement personnel should enter first. Fire and medical personnel enter only after the area is declared safe.
7 Shootings, stabbings, and traumatic suicides are primarily police matters.
8 If the situation deteriorates, leave the building. Meet law enforcement personnel at a secure location and advise them of the situation.
9 A dead paramedic is a useless paramedic.

▼   ▼

8

BARROOM SITUATIONS

Every city has a district that is noted for problems. When the address of the local "Knife and Gun Club" is announced by the dispatcher, everyone hearing the call reacts. Most are thankful that they do not have to respond, but others feel a chill up their spine and a knot in their stomach as they hurry to their unit.

The address may not be a barroom. Difficult situations are also encountered in sophisticated nightclubs, casinos, crowded restaurants, and even churches. Any location with a large gathering of people can create difficulties for fire and rescue personnel.

The problems vary from the potential for extreme personal danger to the ridiculous situation that hinders patient care. For example, while waiting on a table at the height of the dinner hour, a waiter in an expensive restaurant has a heart attack. When the medic crew arrives, they find the waiter in full cardiac arrest on the floor next to a table. While the paramedics work the cardiac arrest victim, waiters step over the patient's legs and the paramedic's equipment, and diners at neighboring tables are enjoying their meal as if nothing had happened.[1]

Consider the danger if this situation occurs in the local knife and gun club establishment. During treatment of the patient, you ask the bartender to turn down the music so that you can take a blood pressure reading. After several moments of quiet, one of the customers begins yelling at the bartender, "Turn the jukebox up, I can't hear the music!"

SIZE UP

Begin *size up* as soon as you receive the call. Your subconscious reaction to the address starts the information-gathering process. Follow your initial reaction to the information received from the dispatcher with a series of questions:

1. Does the establishment have a history of trouble?
   ▶ Have you personally experienced trouble during calls at this address?
   ▶ Did the trouble endanger your life?
   ▶ Did the trouble interfere with patient care?
2. What is the reported nature of the incident?
   ▶ Was the problem incited by natural causes, such as a heart attack?
   ▶ Was the injury accidental or the result of a violent act?
3. If the injury was the result of violence, consider the following:
   ▶ Is the person who caused the injury still at the scene?
   ▶ Is violence still occurring?
4. Are the police responding to this call?
   ▶ Are they at the scene?
   ▶ What is their estimated time of arrival?

Depending on the location of the call, time of day, and nature of the call, many other questions need to be considered. By gathering information about the call during the response, you should have enough facts to make a go or no-go decision when you arrive at the scene. If you are not comfortable with the situation when you arrive, wait for police assistance before entering the establishment.

ENTERING THE ESTABLISHMENT

When you decide to enter the building, use the following tactics to increase your personal safety. If you enter a dimly lighted establishment (such as a barroom) during daylight hours, the instant loss of light may be deadly. To partially compensate for the subdued lighting, close one eye, preferably your strong eye, before getting out of your unit. Keep this eye closed as you approach and enter the building. After you are inside, open it. This eye will be adjusted to less light and will assist you in seeing deeper into the dimness.

Do not look directly at objects or people until both eyes have fully adjusted. At first, you will see more clearly with peripheral vision than with direct observation. To use this technique, do not look directly at the object of concern, but look several degrees off-center. Do not fix your gaze on a single object or person; keep your eyes moving around the main object of interest. This movement will increase your off-center vision while your eyes adjust to the available light.[2]

As soon as the door closes behind you and your partner, step to one side of the entrance, if possible (Figure 8-1). To prevent anyone from get-

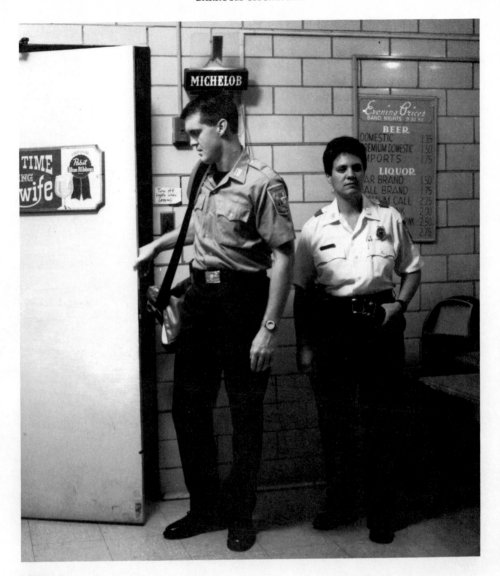

FIGURE 8-1
Before locating the patient, step to the side of the entrance and size up the room.

ting behind you, remain close to the wall. Stay in this position and assess what you see and hear. The decision to proceed farther into the building or withdraw to the parking lot and wait for police support is greatly influenced by your gut feeling about the emotional temperature of the room. Every situation is different—only the people on the scene can make the decision to proceed or withdraw.

Identify the person who called for assistance. In many establishments the bartenders and doormen (bouncers) are the most sober people on the premises. Ask them about the situation. If the patient has been injured in a

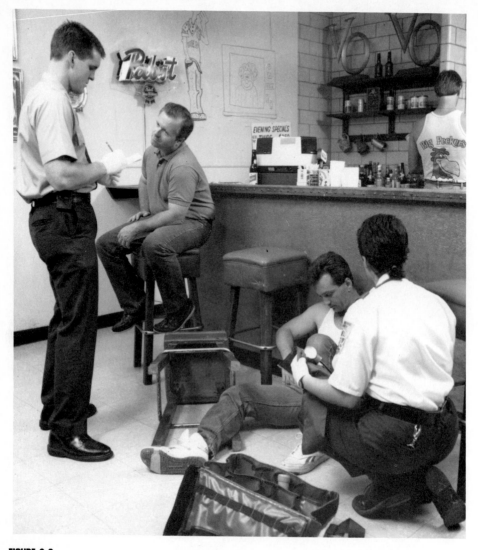

FIGURE 8-2
One medic should stand and observe the emotional temperature of the room while the other medic assesses the patient.

fight, identify who caused the injury. Is that person still in the building? Was a weapon involved? Where is the weapon?

TUNNEL VISION

After the patient is located, do not lose sight of what is happening around you. To prevent the tunnel vision encountered by most emergency medical services personnel while assessing the patient, one medic watches the crowd and the other finds out what needs to be done before the patient can be moved (Figure 8-2). The medic not involved in patient care gathers information about the incident. Remain together during this process; separation may be dangerous for you, your partner, and your patient.

Never touch anyone in the room except the patient. Depending on a patron's state of sobriety, your actions, no matter how innocent, may be interpreted as an act of aggression or a move that will belittle the person in the eyes of friends.

Always be aware of the emotional temperature of the room. If the atmosphere starts to become dangerous, be prepared to move the patient quickly to safety and be clear of the room before an emotional explosion occurs.

THE HASTY RETREAT

In some areas, protocol still emphasizes stabilization and treatment of patients wherever they are found. Emergency service providers that do not strictly follow local protocol may receive disciplinary action ranging from a verbal reprimand to a loss of certification, depending on the seriousness of the violation. More recently the national trend in patient care is toward rapid evaluation, timely transportation, and stabilization en route to the medical care facility.

In some instances, providing patient care in the original location is not practical because of the surroundings. If it will not jeopardize patient care, consider moving the victim out of the public eye. This action will preserve the patient's and the family's dignity.

Anticipate the need to evacuate the patient quickly to an area of safety. If possible, move toward the unit. If not, move to another area within the building or, as a last resort, behind the bar or against a wall to wait for assistance.

Before the days of emergency medical technicians and paramedics, standard procedure was for ambulance personnel to put the victim on a stretcher, place the stretcher in the ambulance, and race for a hospital. They had minimal medical training and were only a fast taxi service. Although current standards indicate rapid assessment, appropriate intervention, and rapid transportation to a proper facility, some situations still justify the old *swoop and scoop* tactics.

Any victim found in a burning building is usually removed to safety before treatment begins. This action is never questioned as a possible violation of protocol. The imminent danger to the victim and the rescuer justifies immediate removal to a safe location (Figure 8-3).

Equally hazardous conditions are found in any public gathering place, especially after the occurrence of a violent act. Treat situations involving violent actions the same way as any other hazardous incident—get in, get the patient, and get out.

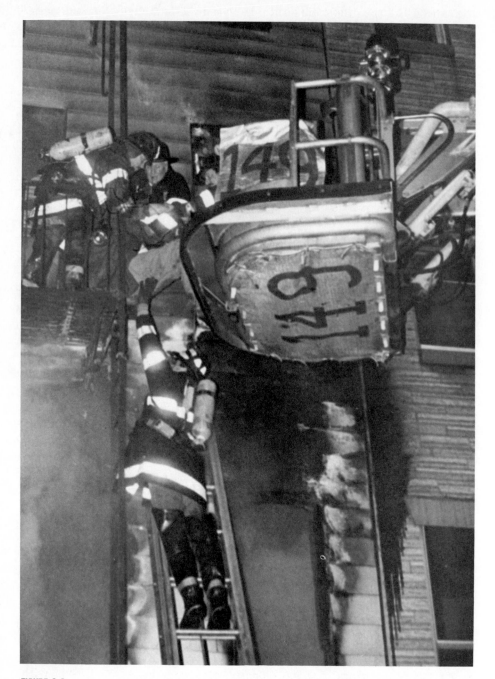

FIGURE 8-3

Treat patients found in violent atmospheres the same way as those found in
burning buildings—remove the patient to a safe location before starting care.
(Courtesy T.W. McNulty, Fire Department of the City of New York, Randall's Island, N.Y.)

In situations where violence suddenly erupts around you, create a diversion by yelling, "Hey, don't throw that!" When your aggressor ducks or turns, run for the door. If possible, take the patient with you.

If the potential for violence is apparent when you enter an establishment, do not stay there. Make a safe retreat by announcing to the room in general, "We need to get the stretcher." Return to the unit and call for police assistance. While waiting for the police to arrive, discuss the situation with your partner, and assemble the equipment you will need to treat the patient. Be ready to enter and start treatment as soon as the police arrive and declare the area safe.

USING AVAILABLE HUMAN RESOURCES

If the crowd becomes unruly and you believe you will have trouble getting the patient to the door, use the *option of last resorts*. Ask the biggest and meanest-looking person, "We need your help in getting the patient through this crowd. Can you move everybody out of our way so we can get out of here?" You are transferring the unmanageable problem of onlooker interference and crowd control to this person. In establishments where the situation deteriorates to where this request is necessary, someone will usually accept the challenge of clearing a path for you. Make sure the person you ask is not the same person who caused the injury to your patient!

▼   **SURVIVAL TIPS**   ▼

1 Remember, the dispatched call may not be what you find when you arrive. The "man choking" in the local restaurant may have been caused by a person's hands around his throat and not because he did not chew his food properly.
2 Never enter a public gathering place without a portable radio. You may need to call for assistance to leave.
3 Never enter a public gathering place alone for a reported trauma injury. Two rescuers should be the minimum number of personnel authorized to initially investigate this type of incident.
4 Never enter an establishment known to be a trouble area without confirming that the police are responding. Do not assume that the dispatcher notified the police at the time of alarm, *always ask!*
5 Never enter an establishment if you believe your safety is in question. Notify the dispatcher that you are remaining outside until the police arrive and allow them to enter the building first.
6 Always document any conditions forcing you to move the patient without proper packaging. Emphasize in your report why this was necessary; for example, "The building was on fire," or "The people were throwing bottles at us."

9

COVER AND CONCEALMENT

Shortly after 4 PM on 18 July 1984, the San Diego Fire Department received a report of a shooting incident at a McDonald's restaurant in San Ysidro. The first responding engine company was forced to stop short of the scene and seek cover behind the engine because of gunfire. The responding battalion chief stopped about 30 yards behind the engine and used his vehicle for cover until the scene was secured by the police department (Figure 9-1).[1]

When approaching an incident, train yourself to scan the area quickly for objects that you can use for protection if violence unexpectedly erupts. Make this action a subconscious procedure that identifies potential locations of cover or concealment. Maintain an awareness of your immediate surroundings so that when an attack occurs, you can instinctively locate a safe area. If you fail to react instantly to a sudden attack, you may be seriously injured or killed.

Never assume you will not be harmed because you are clearly identified as a member of the fire department or an EMS responder. Always assume the person with the gun will shoot anyone in sight. If the police seek cover, you must not remain in the immediate vicinity of the operation (Figure 9-2).

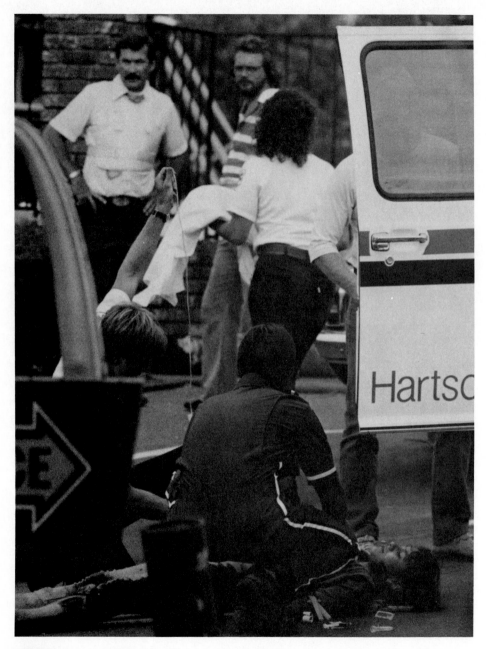

FIGURE 9-1
Medical personnel treat victim of a massacre at McDonald's restaurant in San Ysidro, California. *(Courtesy Union-Tribune Publishing Co., San Diego.)*

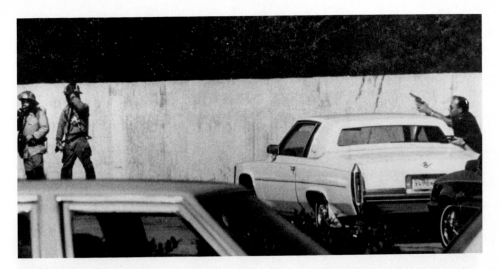

FIGURE 9-2
The state-of-the-art protective clothing worn by the firefighters standing on the left protects them from heat, not bullets. The police officer would be safer behind the engine block or wheel area. *(Courtesy The Tampa Tribune, Tampa, Fla.)*

COVER

Recognize the difference between objects that provide cover and those that offer concealment only. Objects that are usually impenetrable to bullets include trees, utility poles, mail-collection boxes, dumpsters, curbs, vehicles, and depressions in the ground and are considered as cover. When you are using cover, make your body conform to the shape of the object as much as possible (Figure 9-3). For example, if you crouch behind a mail-collection box, you are protected from the knees up, but the person that is firing at you can see your ankles and feet. If any part of your body is exposed, it can be hit. To minimize exposure, place your feet behind the posts that support the mailbox (Figure 9-4).

If your assailant is on higher ground than you (such as in an upper-floor window or on a roof), the aggressor can see the upper part of your torso or head over the top of your cover, especially if you are using a wall or motor vehicle as cover (Figure 9-5).

Use the engine block and wheel area of a motor vehicle as cover (see Chapter 2). Avoid the area near the fuel tank, and do not use the area between the wheels as cover. Even though the aggressor cannot see you in this position, a skilled shot can hit you by ricochetting bullets off of the pavement in front of your position. Bullets do not bounce off solid objects at the same angle at which they initially hit. When a bullet hits a hard surface (such as a concrete wall or pavement), it flattens out and travels parallel to the surface at an angle far less than the angle of aim (Figure 9-6).[2] During the Texas Tower incident in 1966, an ambulance driver was lying behind the ambulance in the area between the wheels when the assailant

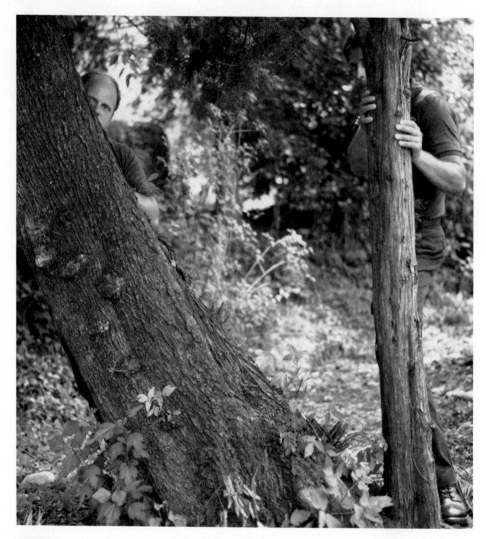

FIGURE 9-3
Pick a tree that is large enough to conceal all of your body.

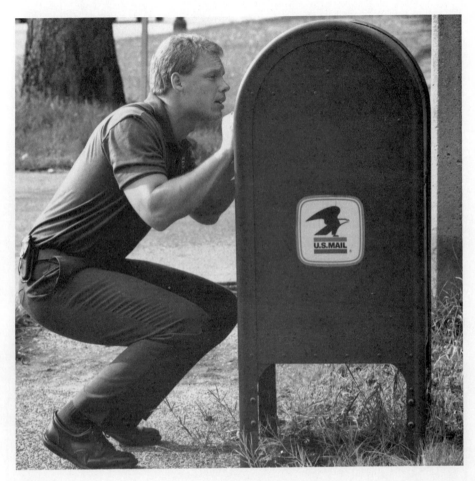

FIGURE 9-4
A large, blue mailbox on a corner provides cover; the one on a post in front of your house does not.

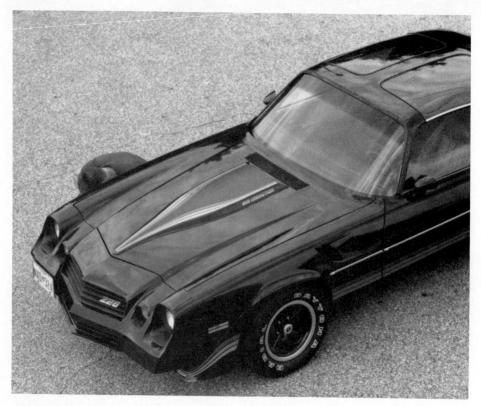

FIGURE 9-5
Assailant can see part of your body from above your position of cover.

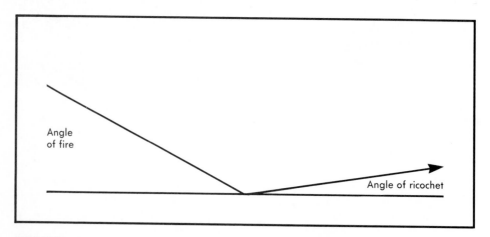

FIGURE 9-6
The ricochet's angle is much less than that of the original shot.

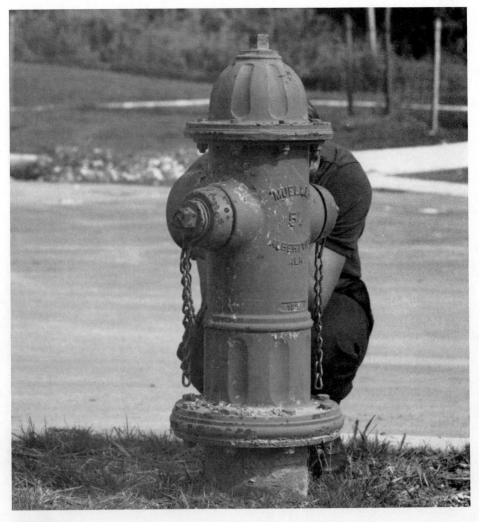

FIGURE 9-7
Fire hydrants provide excellent cover from bullets, but hiding behind one becomes uncomfortable quickly.

purposely fired at the ground on the opposite side of the medic unit. The bullets traveled under the unit and struck and killed the driver.

Select a fire hydrant as cover only if no larger objects are immediately available. You will soon become uncomfortable trying to conform your body to such a small object. You will probably be shot in the arm, knee, or shoulder, but if this is the only cover available, it is better than remaining in the open (Figure 9-7).

Items inside a structure and the structure itself can provide cover or concealment. Make sure that the item you choose for cover can stop a bullet. Use a solid oak desk or a refrigerator. If you dive behind the sofa or a stuffed chair, you have concealed yourself but are not protected by cover.

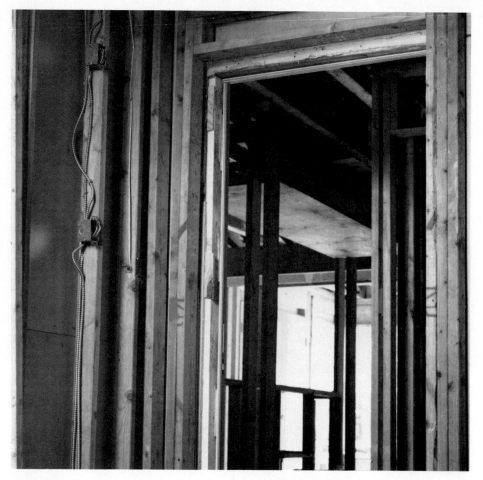

FIGURE 9-8
The density of wall framing is greater near doors and windows.

USING WALLS AS COVER

Many walls look as if they will provide safe cover but, because of their material, will provide only concealment. For your safety and survival, you must recognize if the type of wall you have chosen gives you cover or concealment only. For example, brick or concrete-block walls are much safer than cinder-block walls because of the porous nature of cinder blocks. Interior walls constructed with wood or aluminum studs and covered with drywall, lath and plaster, or siding conceal you but are not good cover because they are not impenetrable. If you seek protection behind a frame wall, try to stand near the door or window frames. These areas are usually constructed with extra framing materials that contain more wood than other areas of the wall (Figure 9-8).

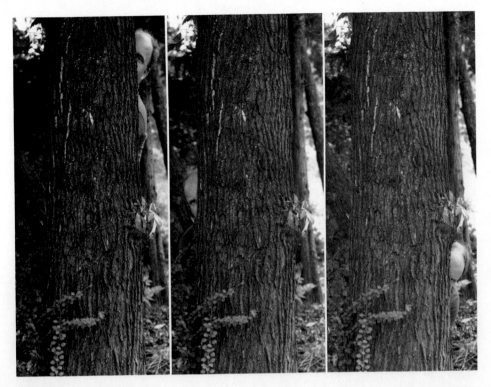

FIGURE 9-9
If you must analyze your position, look from a different height and angle each time.

BODY POSITION

Whenever possible, choose cover that permits you to stand. If you are trapped for a long time, standing is the most comfortable and versatile position. You can shift your body slightly without exposing yourself and change your location quickly when the need arises.

If you cannot stand because of the cover or the assailant's position, squat rather than sit, and sit rather than lie. The prone position is the most difficult for safely changing positions or locations.

CHANGING LOCATIONS

Change locations only if the new location is better cover, it is farther from the hostile atmosphere, and you can move without revealing yourself to the assailant. Do not change your position of cover just for the sake of changing.

To evaluate the advisability of changing locations, quickly look out from your cover (Figure 9-9). Look from a different height and angle each

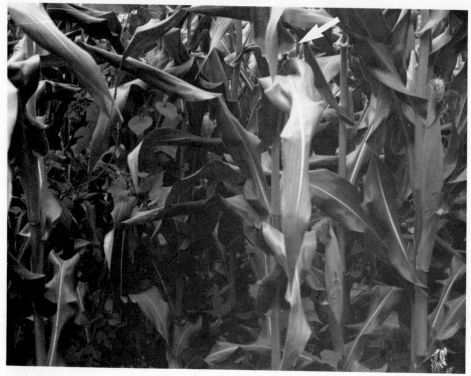

FIGURE 9-10
A man standing in a cornfield is practically invisible.

time. Use the "quick-peek" technique and return to cover as quickly as possible.

If you decide that you would be safer in another location, do not run directly away from the assailant's position; run in a zig-zag pattern. You have much less chance of being hit if your movement takes you across the assailant's field of view.

CONCEALMENT

Tall grass, shrubbery, and dark shadows are considered areas of concealment. When cover is not readily available, use concealment to provide some protection while you assess your position and seek cover.

Areas of concealment are more available after dark than during daylight hours. If you are involved in a violent situation at night, move into the darkness and stand still. The assailant cannot see you and may not shoot. If shots are fired randomly, chances are you will not be hit.

Jumping into tall grass or a cornfield will conceal you from your assailant day or night (Figure 9-10). Remain motionless so that the foliage does not move. After you have analyzed the situation, move toward cover.

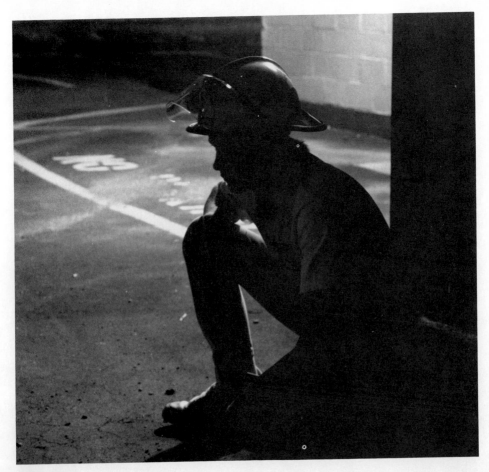

FIGURE 9-11
Do not stand between a light and your assailant.

▼   **SURVIVAL TIPS**   ▼

1   Unless you *know* the thickness and quality of material used in the construction of interior walls and furnishings, treat the objects as concealment.
2   When concealed, you cannot be seen by your assailant, but you can be heard. Move as quietly as possible.
3   If you are concealed from view behind a large bush or in a dark shadow, you may feel secure, but if a streetlight is behind you or an approaching vehicle silhouettes you in the headlights, you are again visible (Figure 9-11).

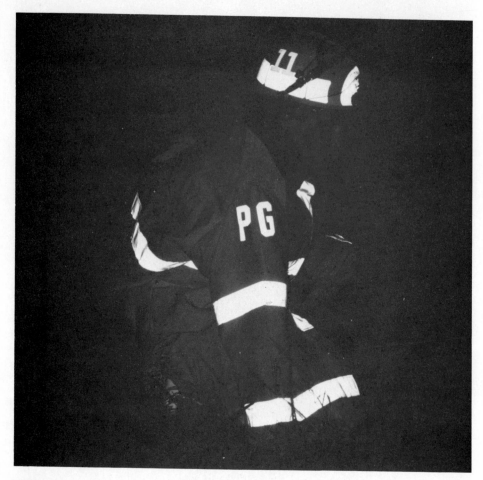

FIGURE 9-12
If not for the reflective tape, this firefighter would be invisible.

4 Do not look out from your cover to see what is happening. Until the area is secured, any hostile incident is a law enforcement problem. Remain completely concealed from the assailant until you hear the all-clear signal.

5 Before you use darkness as concealment, remove all clothing with reflective tape. In cold temperatures or inclement weather, wear the garments inside out to protect you from the elements (Figure 9-12).

10

HOSTAGE SITUATIONS

On 28 May 1982, in Montgomery County, Maryland, a man crashed his car through the north entrance of the IBM building and ran through the building, randomly firing a machine gun at occupants.[1] Firefighters and paramedics arrived before SWAT personnel and entered the building. SWAT personnel, equipped with flak vests, M-16s, and tear gas, relieved the first rescue squad, who had only jump kits and good intentions. After the fire chief was told about the nature of the incident, all fire department personnel (except the SWAT medics) were withdrawn from the building until the SWAT team had secured the building and declared the area safe. When the 7-hour incident ended, approximately 200 people had been treated or undergone triage—3 died (Figure 10-1).

Fire and EMS personnel sometimes arrive on a scene before it is secure. When law enforcement personnel arrive, they may try to include paramedics as members of the initial entry team.[2] If you have not been trained for this type of operation, do not participate in the assault on the aggressor's position (Figure 10-2). Without preparation, emergency response personnel are thrust into circumstances that offer the possibility of personal injury or becoming a hostage themselves. Hostage situations are law enforcement problems until the scene is secure (Figure 10-3).

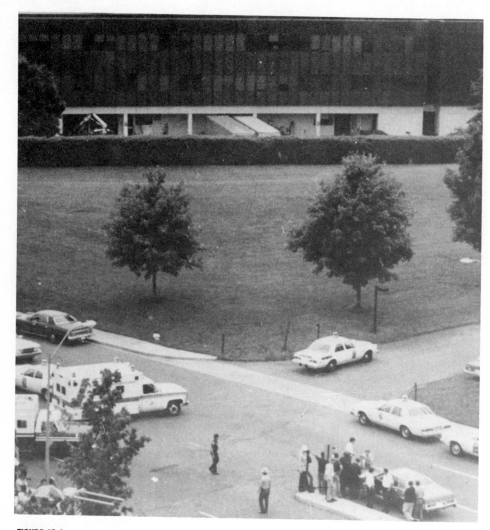

FIGURE 10-1
Police and rescue workers assembled outside IBM building. *(Courtesy Wide World Photos, New York.)*

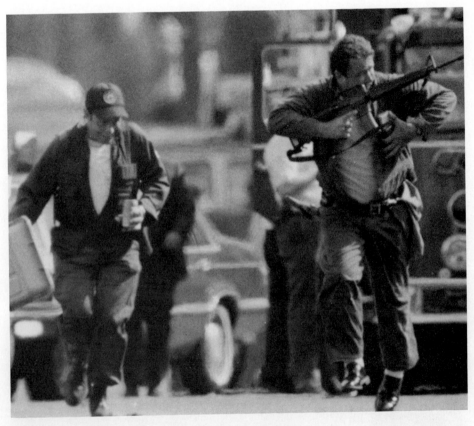

FIGURE 10-2
While fire department personnel remain in a secure staging area, law enforcement personnel change positions. *(Courtesy The Phila. Inquirer, Philadelphia.)*

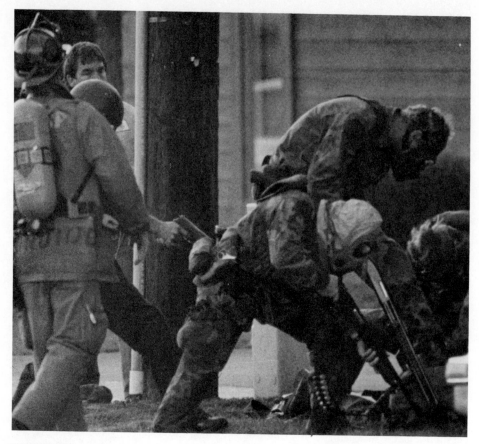

FIGURE 10-3
Fire, rescue, and EMS personnel must remain behind the police-barricade line until the area is secure. Would you consider this area secure? *(Courtesy Union-Tribune Publishing Co., San Diego.)*

SURVIVING AS A HOSTAGE

Have you considered what you will do if you meet an armed adversary? No rules apply; anything can happen depending on the assailant, your position, and your reactions.

The possibility of being taken hostage is extremely remote, but it does exist. If you are taken hostage, remember that most hostage incidents in the United States last between 4½ and 5 hours. Certain ways you behave will greatly enhance your chances of surviving the ordeal unscathed.[3]

Hostages are usually held as a form of human collateral to ensure compliance with a promise made by someone charged with the responsibility of securing the hostages' freedom.[4] You increase your chances of survival as a hostage if you anticipate the feelings and actions of the hostage taker and the people attempting to gain your release. Statistics indicate that if you remain calm, you have a 95% chance of surviving physically unharmed.[5]

The psychological problems that develop are of greater concern than the possible physical abuse. Even if you are physically unharmed, expect to experience some psychological problems during the incident, especially after the situation ends. A person held hostage needs professional counseling after the release to prevent long-term problems later. If you know what to expect as a hostage, you may have fewer psychological problems during the situation and after your release.

PEOPLE WHO TAKE HOSTAGES

Hostage takers are classified as *crazies, criminals,* or *crusaders.*

Crazies: People that are mentally disturbed are involved in 52% of all hostage incidents.[6] A spouse, children, other relatives, or friends may be taken hostage. The mentally disturbed are rarely predictable and usually operate by a set of rules known only to themselves. Their reasons for taking hostages may be real or imagined. According to the FBI, these people typically fall into one of these diagnostic categories: paranoid schizophrenic, manic-depressive illness (depressed type), antisocial personality, or inadequate personality.[7]

Criminals: A criminal will take hostages to gain freedom from an unexpected entrapment. The hostages are usually people who are at the scene of the crime when something goes wrong. Consider the following situation:

You stop the medic unit at a local convenience store to buy ice cream. The driver remains with the unit, and you enter the store and find a robbery in progress. The robber sees your uniform and the light bar on top of the unit. Instant panic! In the would-be robber's eyes, you are a cop—and the robber is in big trouble. You are suddenly taken hostage along with everyone else in the store.

Crusaders: Crusaders are terrorists. They may be social activists, revolutionaries such as neo-Nazi organizations, or a local chapter of a motorcycle gang. We do not like to think that these groups operate in our area, but they do, and their presence continues to grow. Extreme left-wing, right-wing, radical-religious, single-issue, or hate groups are found throughout the nation. Organizations including the Ku Klux Klan, the United Freedom Front, the Armed Resistance Unit, and the May 19 Organization operate within our borders daily. Terrorist groups from West Germany, Italy, and the Middle East import violence into the United States. In 1985 the FBI uncovered a plot to assassinate the prime minister of India while he was in our country. The same year, they stopped a pro-Libyan organization from carrying out three assassinations in the United States. Recently a person with ties to a Middle East group placed three homemade bombs along the New Jersey Turnpike.[8]

Of the three classifications of hostage takers, you are least likely to encounter terrorists. Their activities are well planned and precisely executed. However, you may be involved in terrorist activities. If government offices, military installations, nuclear power plants, defense contractors, research facilities, and dams are in your area, you are susceptible to the threat. According to the International Association of Chiefs of Police (1978), only complete familiarization with and preparation for terrorism can equip anyone to survive a confrontation with dignity.[9]

STAGES OF A HOSTAGE SITUATION

The six stages involved in taking and maintaining hostages are outlined in the box. Emergency services workers taken hostage are most affected by the capture, transport, and holding stages.

Capture Stage

When an emergency services worker is taken hostage, the hostage taker is as surprised as the person being captured. The mentally disturbed and criminals rarely plan this action, but if it happens, they may use the hostage as a medium of exchange or as a shield for the hostage-taker's safety and escape.[10]

The hostage taker is extremely nervous and trying to gain control of what has suddenly become an unsettled situation. At this stage, you are in grave personal danger. Assume that the person on the other end of the gun will use violence if you do not follow instructions.

Do not attempt to escape. If your escape attempt fails, what will your new position be with your abductor? Consider the safety of any other hostages. If your actions antagonize your captor, your chances of being hurt increase. You must avoid personal injury, remain calm, and control the instinctive anger that occurs when you are physically abused.

At the moment of capture, you may feel that it is all a bad dream because your mind cannot adjust quickly to a radical change. The automatic defense of denial facilitates the transition from being in control of your surroundings to acknowledging your defenselessness.[11]

SIX STAGES OF A HOSTAGE SITUATION

Stage 1 - *Surveillance* The terrorist group identifies and watches the intended hostage until every move is known. The terrorist learns as much about the intended hostage as possible before making the capture.

Stage 2 - *Capture* The hostage taker is usually excited, armed, and capable of violent actions.

Stage 3 - *Transport* The group moves the hostage to a different location within the same general area.

Stage 4 - *Holding* Negotiations have begun for your release; the strain of waiting may affect you psychologically.

Stage 5 - *Move* You are transported to a different location.

Stage 6 - *Resolution* You are released after successful negotiations or an assault on the hostage-taker's position by SWAT members.

Transport Stage

You may be transported from where you are taken hostage to where the hostage taker feels more secure. This move may be only to the other side of the room or to another part of the same building.

If you are transported soon after capture, the aggressor will still be agitated. During this stage, expect to receive harsh commands from your captor. If the captor feels you are moving too slowly, expect physical abuse such as pushing, dragging, or kicking.

If the abductor has time, you may be tied, gagged, and blindfolded before being transported. Your body may slip into shock, and if you have been slow in following instructions, you will experience physical pain and emotional instability. Your perceptions may be distorted, especially if you are blindfolded.

At this time you must regain your composure. With preparation and pre-planning, you can reduce the shock of this experience and recover your senses quickly. Collect as much information as possible about your location. Concentrate! What do you hear? Are church bells ringing? Do you hear trains, airplanes, or street traffic? Are people talking in a foreign language? Do you smell animals, chemicals, or food? If you used stairs, try to remember the number of floors. Did you leave the original building? If you are transported by vehicle, analyze the route of travel. Count the number, the direction, and the order of turns. Be aware of outside noises that will help reconstruct the route. Note the number of captors involved and the types and quantity of weapons. The more you can remember about the transport stage of your captivity, the more help you will be to the law enforcement agencies after your release.

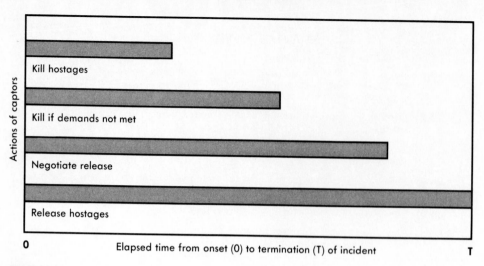

FIGURE 10-4
Thresholds of hostage safety.

Holding Stage

During the holding stage, you begin to develop psychological and emotional problems. The situation has calmed slightly, and law enforcement is at the scene and negotiating for your release. The holding stage is tedious; you sit, wait, and hope for a safe release. Hostage negotiators count on time to bring an incident to a safe and successful conclusion. Your chances of survival increase proportionally from the time of your capture to the time of your release.[12] In the beginning stages, your captor usually says, "I'm going to kill you!" but you are kept alive so that the demands will be met (Figure 10-4).

Even if negotiations have started, do not predict an exact time or date of release. If you set an unrealistic goal (such as 4 hours) and are wrong, you will feel demoralized. Only your abductors decide when you will be released. If you have been captured by terrorists, plan for a much longer time in captivity than if your captors were criminals or mentally disturbed. Accept the fact that you have no control over when you will be freed.

During this stage your mental state is a greater danger to you than your captors are. After you reach the holding area, your captors will try to break your spirit. You may be forced to ask for food and permission to sleep and use the toilet.[13]

Manage yourself and your personal environment. Do not do anything that will attract unwanted attention, and do not stare at your captors. If you convincingly fake a heart attack or sickness, you become less valuable to your captors. If they feel you are starting to get in their way or on their nerves, they may kill you. Any one of your captors can walk in and kill you at any time. Your only chance to stay alive is in your role as a bargaining chip. Do not pressure or agitate them into changing their plans. Be espe-

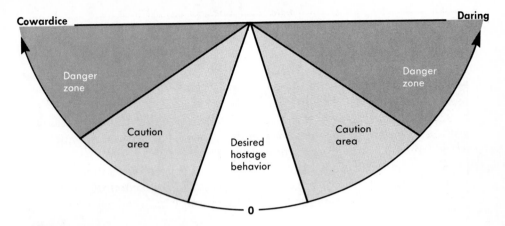

FIGURE 10-5
Behavior continuum model.

cially careful of female hostage takers. They are usually easy to anger and quicker to use violence.

Hostage negotiators suggest you find a middle ground between being too daring and being a coward. A behavior continuum model (Figure 10-5) illustrates the danger zones and caution areas of your actions.

Because you are wearing a uniform, other hostages may look to you for guidance and strength. Your captors may consider this image of authority as a threat. Anything that draws attention to you increases the possibility of violence. Make every effort to be inconspicuous. Develop a nonthreatening image by removing the badge, collar pins, and patches from your uniform, or turn your uniform shirt inside out so these items are not visible.

Sometimes you will have to ignore your modesty. If you are given the opportunity to bathe or use bathroom facilities, do it, regardless of the presence of male or female guards or other hostages.

Meals may be provided only once a day. When you are given food, divide it into three portions for breakfast, lunch, and supper. Try to maintain a normal, daily routine.

As your time in captivity increases, exercise becomes increasingly important to your physical and mental conditioning. Vietnam prisoners exercised, even when they were confined to a small box—a contributing factor to their survival.

Keeping your mind active is as important as physical exercise. Write letters (even if they will not be mailed), read anything you can find, and fantasize—time will pass more easily under adverse conditions.

Measure time by the meals, the guard's behavior (for example, sleepy at night), and outside noises (birds in the morning, crickets at night). Keep a calendar of days and celebrate special events such as holidays and birthdays. Establish a daily routine for meals, personal hygiene, housekeeping your own space, rest, exercise, and sleeping periods.

THE STOCKHOLM SYNDROME

On 23 August 1973, four employees of the Sveriges Kreditbank in Stockholm, Sweden, were taken hostage during an attempted bank robbery. They were held by their captors for 131 hours. During the incident the hostages became more afraid of the police than the robbers.[14] This feeling became known as the "Stockholm Syndrome."

Identifying with captors is a psychological reaction to circumstances that force you to mentally fight for your life. Even after witnessing your abductors commit unspeakable crimes against others, your survival instinct tells you that your captors must think of you as a friendly and cooperative person. Because you are not directly experiencing discomfort, you may think, "These people are not so bad; I understand what they are doing, and I feel they are right."

The Stockholm Syndrome also affects the hostage taker. A captor who becomes friendly with hostages will not readily harm or kill them. After the hostage taker interacts with the hostages, chances are less that you will be the victim of aggressive action. Terrorist organizations know the danger of this happening. If you notice different people guarding you, realize that a dangerous situation may be developing. To prevent human contact between guards and hostages, some organizations require guards to wear hoods to negate the effect of face-to-face contact.

For this syndrome to develop, positive contact between the hostages and the hostage takers must take place. The length of time required before the syndrome begins to form is undetermined. Humane actions by the hostage takers, such as allowing the hostages to use toilet facilities, giving them blankets when it is cold, or talking with them on a personal level, are signs that a relationship is beginning. The hostages will start to look at their captors as humans with problems similar to their own and may blame law enforcement personnel for their continued imprisonment. If the hostage takers subject the hostages to beatings, pain, dehumanizing living conditions, or other forms of negative association during their time in captivity, the syndrome will not develop.[15]

LAW ENFORCEMENT PROCEDURES IN A HOSTAGE SITUATION

Most modern law enforcement agencies either have or have access to a highly trained negotiating team. The number of members assigned to the team, the agencies represented, and the professional background of team members vary by jurisdiction. The one thing they all have in common is that the safety of the hostages is the primary concern.

Until the negotiating team arrives on the scene, law enforcement personnel and your captors may have no contact. Law enforcement officers recognize the value of time in a hostage situation. At the beginning of an incident involving hostages, emotions are usually high, and all of the participants are thinking and acting emotionally rather than rationally.[16] As time passes, the situation becomes less tense for all persons involved, including the police.

Whenever possible, negotiators should not attempt any contact with the hostage takers until the incident seems stabilized. The negotiators gather information about the hostages and the hostage takers during this waiting period. The negotiators will probably be talking with your captors by telephone instead of face-to-face. The telephone ensures a private conversation and the safety of the negotiating parties.

Remember, after all demands for release or surrender have been met, the hostage taker will probably not escape successfully. Stay away from doors and windows. After your captors have tried to escape or surrendered to the police, stay where you are. Do not leave the area where you were being held until you are told to do so by law enforcement personnel. If the police assault your location in an attempted rescue, lie on the floor and place your hands on your head. Remain in that position until your rescuers tell you to move.

The time immediately after your rescue is just as critical to your safety as when you were first captured. The rescuers will not recognize you as a hostage but will treat everyone in the room as a suspect. You must control your emotions and follow the rescuer's instructions completely. After you have been properly identified and the area is declared safe, you will have time to thank your rescuers.

▼ SURVIVAL TIPS ▼

1 Maintain your composure and remain calm.
2 Follow your captor's instructions completely.
3 Inform your captors of any medical problems. If you require scheduled medication, you may be released.
4 Do not stare at your captors. Be as inconspicuous as possible and do not make any sudden moves.
5 Accept the fact that you are a hostage. When you talk with your captors, do not antagonize them—talk in your normal voice.
6 Do not fight sleep. Resting is one way of reducing anxiety.
7 Accept any favors offered by your abductors, including food, beverages, and toilet privileges.
8 Do not try to overpower your captors. Failure will cause violent and possibly fatal reactions.
9 Stay clear of doors and windows. If law enforcement personnel make an assault on your position, lie flat on the floor and remain motionless until you are instructed to move.
10 To prevent lasting emotional trauma, accept psychological counseling after a hostage experience.

11

BOMBS, BOOBY TRAPS, AND MAKESHIFT WEAPONS

You may encounter illegal bombs, booby traps, and other makeshift weapons when least expected. The location or nature of the call could indicate the need for extra caution based on previous incidents. Never assume that a harmless-looking package, a usually safe area, or a calm, friendly individual will not present a threat. These threats can be as seemingly harmless as an old war relic in your home or station. For example, if not properly disarmed, a Civil War cannonball or a World War II grenade can be deadly.

WHO USES EXPLOSIVES?

Many civilian and military occupations require the use of explosives. Companies that build roads, demolish buildings, and perform mining operations need them for their daily routine. Whenever you respond to a location where these activities are occurring or have occurred, proceed with extra caution.

Some organizations use explosives illegally. These groups include radicals, criminals, psychotics, pyromaniacs, rival labor groups, terrorists, and professional saboteurs. You may also have to deal with children experimenting with explosives.[1]

Illegal users may protect their operation by using booby traps. Because of the increased crime rate, many law-abiding small-business owners are il-

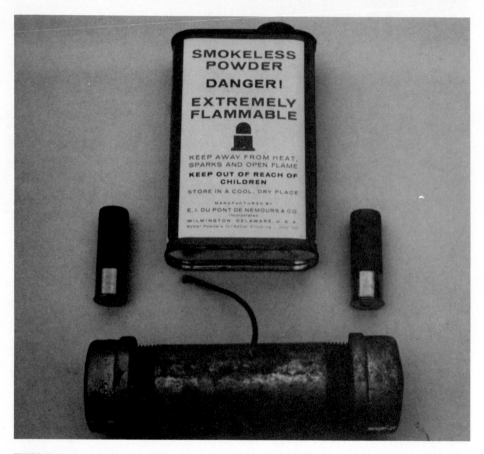

FIGURE 11-1

Low explosives are designed to propel bullets, but when confined in a pipe bomb, they can be deadly.

legally installing booby traps to protect their property. Remember that anyone can use makeshift weapons, which can range from an umbrella used in anger to a carefully constructed pipe bomb used with the intent to kill.

BOMBS AND EXPLOSIVES

From 1977 to 1986, 24,677 explosive incidents were reported to the Bureau of Alcohol, Tobacco, and Firearms.[2] In these incidents, 757 persons were killed and 3913 injured. These numbers justify the importance of emergency services personnel becoming familiar with different kinds of explosives.

Explosives are generally classified as *low explosives, primary high explosives,* or *secondary high explosives.* Low explosives (such as black powder and rifle powder) are the most readily available and are usually preferred by psychotics and saboteurs (Figure 11-1).[3] Low explosives burn

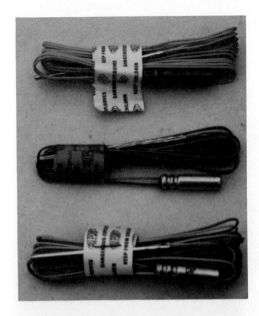

FIGURE 11-2
Blasting caps are approximately
¼-inch in diameter and 1 to 6 inches
long. A copper or aluminum case is
closed at one end and contains a
measured amount of primary high
explosives.

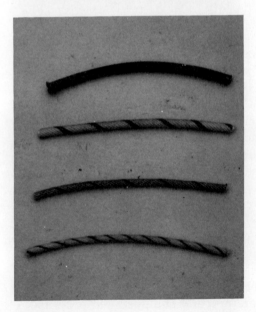

FIGURE 11-3
Detonating cords, unlike blasting
caps, are not sensitive to heat, shock,
or friction.

suddenly and violently at speeds up to 400 m/s and produce pressures of
approximately 30,000 psi.[4]

Primers and *detonators* are the two major types of primary high explosives. Blasting caps, which are used to detonate the main explosive
charge, are initiated with an electrical signal or a burning time fuse (Figure
11-2). Because blasting caps are extremely sensitive to heat, shock, and
friction, their distribution is under tight control, but some are stolen from
construction sites and authorized storage areas for illegal use.[5]

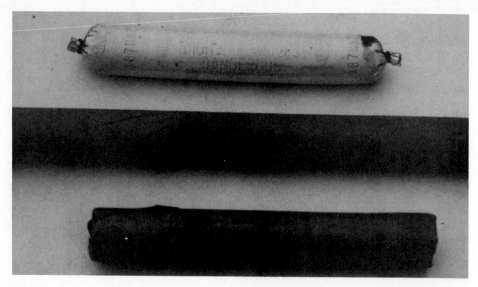

FIGURE 11-4
Secondary high explosives.

Detcord or Primacord transmits the detonating wave from the initiating source to the main charge. It is a strong, flexible cord with a ¼-inch diameter and a center core containing primary high explosives (Figure 11-3).

Secondary high explosives (such as dynamite and TNT) are relatively insensitive to heat, shock, and friction (Figure 11-4). Small, unconfined quantities of these explosives will usually burn instead of exploding when exposed to fire. When detonated, they produce as much as 1 million psi of pressure and travel at a speed of 1000 m/s to 8500 m/s.[6]

Personnel at the scene of a confirmed incident involving explosives or reported bomb scare must have a working knowledge of proper operating procedures. Jurisdictions that have control over incidents involving bombs or other explosives need to develop protocols for a reported or suspected bomb, a confirmed explosive device, and postexplosion operations. Personnel must not participate in any incident involving explosives until they have been thoroughly trained and are properly equipped and protected. If you are not, stop the operation. After all prerequisites have been met, continue the operation with *extreme caution.*

REPORTED OR SUSPECTED BOMB IN THE AREA

You may be asked to assist in searching for an explosive. Unless you are a member of an organization officially assigned to search for reported bombs or explosive devices (such as the Prince Georges County Maryland Fire Department[7]), do not participate in the operation; it is a law enforce-

BOMB THREAT GUIDE

Place this card under telephone

COMPLETE DURING CALL

Questions to ask caller:
1. When is the bomb going to explode?
   _____
2. Where is it located? _____
   _____
3. What does it look like? _____
   _____
4. What kind of bomb is it?_____
   _____
5. What will cause it to explode? _____
   _____
6. Did you place the bomb? _____
   _____
7. Why?_____
   _____
8. What is your address?_____
   _____
9. What is your name?_____

Exact wording of the threat:

_____
_____
_____
_____
_____

Immediately report call to:

_____
_____

Time received: _____
Sex of caller: _____

Front

COMPLETE AFTER CALL

Caller's voice:

____ Calm	____ Nasal
____ Angry	____ Stuttering
____ Excited	____ Lisping
____ Slow	____ Raspy
____ Rapid	____ Deep
____ Soft	____ Ragged
____ Loud	____ Clearing
____ Laughing	throat
____ Crying	____ Deep
____ Normal	breathing
____ Distinct	____ Cracking
____ Slurred	voice
____ Accented	____ Familiar

If the voice is familiar, whom did it
sound like? _____

Background sounds:

____ Street	____ Factory
noises	machines
____ Crockery	____ Animals
____ Voices	____ Clear
____ PA System	____ Static
____ Music	____ Coins dropping
____ Children	(pay phone)
____ Motor	Other_____
____ Office	_____

Threat language:

____ Well spoken	____ Foul
____ Irrational	____ Taped
____ Incoherent	____ Repeating

Back

ment problem. Do not volunteer to assist in searching for an unknown deadly device because of the pressure of the moment.

If a local protocol designates you as the first responder to a bomb scare and you are not trained or equipped to search for a bomb, confirm with dispatch at the time of response that the proper authorities (usually the bomb squad) have been dispatched.

As soon as you arrive on the scene, locate a knowledgeable representative from the area and gather predetermined information that will be useful to the bomb squad. A form that outlines pertinent questions to ask needs to be developed and distributed throughout the business and government community to everyone that receives incoming telephone calls. The two-sided form shown is similar to one provided to all government agencies in Hillsborough County, Florida.

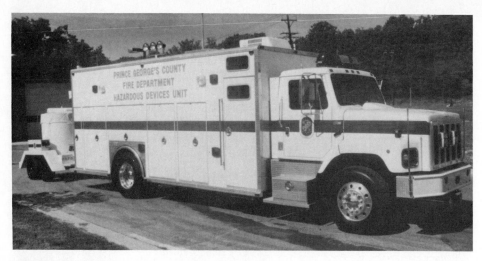

FIGURE 11-5
Hazardous Devices Unit, Prince Georges County Fire Department, Maryland.

The expected time of the explosion and the location of the device are the most important factors when dealing with explosives. If time permits, obtain floor plans of the building and reproduce them on a copying machine in a nearby building so that all search teams have plans of their assigned search areas. Use fire department prefire plans to locate utility shutoffs.

To reduce the possibility of panic, evacuate the building using the pretext of a fire drill. Do not tell the occupants the true nature of the emergency until the evacuation is complete. When evacuating people from schools and commercial and government buildings, keep them at least 150 yards from the area, with 300 yards being the preferred distance.[8] After the building is evacuated, withdraw to a staging area outside of the evacuated area and stand by for the arrival of the bomb squad.

CONDUCTING THE SEARCH

Professional personnel that are highly trained and properly equipped to handle an explosive device should conduct all bomb searches (Figure 11-5). If you do not possess the qualifications, do not participate in the search; remain in the staging area.

CONFIRMED EXPLOSIVE DEVICE

After an explosive device is discovered, fire, rescue, and EMS personnel must remain outside the evacuated area until the device is declared safe or detonated. Personnel who remove or disarm a device do not need or want any unsolicited assistance or advice. They must have total control of the situation and the full cooperation of all emergency services personnel on the scene. If the device detonates unexpectedly, you will need all of your personnel to control the situation. If fire, rescue, or EMS personnel are in the danger zone when the device explodes, they become part of the problem instead of part of the solution. They cannot perform their duties if they are victims of an explosion.

Companies operating at construction sites must be aware of any storage of explosives on the site. If fire involves such an area, evacuate the area and allow it to burn after the life hazard is removed.

POSTEXPLOSION OPERATIONS

Standard operating procedures should dictate the protocol for interagency cooperation at the scene of an explosion. In addition to state and local law enforcement agencies, the FBI and the Bureau of Alcohol, Tobacco, and Firearms may be involved. Each agency will be concerned about a specific phase of the investigation and will be asking the first responders for information.

Do not enter the area of detonation until it has been declared safe. Triage must wait; do not commit personnel to an unstable area for rescue. The building may have more than one device or be in imminent danger of collapse because of the explosion.

Each person entering the area of detonation must be identified. A controlled single point of entry into and out of the area must be established quickly. Someone with the appropriate level of authority to limit access to the area should be assigned to this location to record all personnel movement on a sign-in sheet, which should include the name, the agency represented, a work telephone number, the time in, and the time out. Make this information part of the official incident report.

Take notes on your observations and actions. Do not disturb the area any more than absolutely necessary during rescue and firefighting operations. Do not move dead bodies until told to do so by the authority having jurisdiction over the scene.

BOOBY TRAPS

You may encounter booby traps when least expected. If the police are standing outside the building when you arrive, check with the OIC to make sure the area is secure before entering. If the police are not on the scene and the nature of the call indicates a possible danger, proceed with extreme caution.

Firefighters arriving on the scene of a fire in a residence were advised by police not to enter the structure. This advice was based on the police department's past experience with the occupant. The firefighters controlled

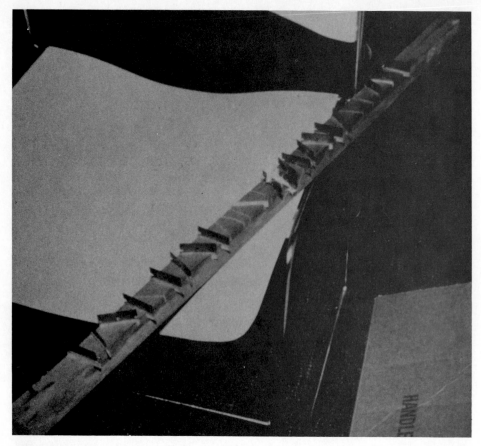

FIGURE 11-6
Board embedded with razor blades used to booby trap windows in a residence.
(Courtesy William S. Ennis, Sr, West Carrollton Division of Fire, West Carrollton, Ohio.)

and extinguished a living room fire from outside the residence and then waited until the bomb squad arrived on the scene.[9]

Many booby traps were found throughout the house, including a hand grenade attached to the back door and ready to explode when the door was opened from the outside (the usual point of entry for an interior attack on a fire in the front part of a house). Every windowsill in the house had 1-inch by 2-inch strips of wood embedded with razor blades attached to the inside of the sill so that people coming through the window would severely cut their hands (Figure 11-6).

Because police department personnel were on the scene before the fire department and were familiar with the occupant of the residence, injuries were prevented. If the fire department had arrived on the scene first, the results would have been devastating.

The purpose of deadly devices is usually not to harm an emergency services worker, but once in place, there is no way to control who will be the victim. A careless step or movement of an object may lead to death or serious injury.

When you work on a patient in questionable surroundings (such as in a "biker house" or "drug house"), be careful what you touch, pick up, or move. Normal-looking household items are often used to rig a booby trap.

MAKESHIFT WEAPONS

Weapons come in many shapes and sizes; the weapons that are the most deadly may not look like weapons. After a weapon is activated, it is usually too late to avoid an injury.

The harmless-looking fountain pen shown in Figure 11-7, A becomes a deadly weapon when the shirt clip is depressed and expels a spring-loaded, sharp rod from the end of the pen (Figure 11-7, B).

Many weapons are designed to be concealed under articles of clothing or disguised to look like a harmless accessory. When the key ring shown in Figure 11-8, A is unscrewed, it becomes a knife (Figure 11-8, B).

Explosives can be concealed in many innocent-looking products. A pipe bomb is inside a toothpaste container in Figure 11-9. The cigarette lighter in Figure 11-10 is an antipersonnel weapon designed to hold explosives. After the fuse is lighted, the device is thrown at the intended victim.

Thoroughly search patients removed from correctional facilities and police stations for weapons before transporting. Your search may reveal something as innocent-looking as a bar of soap in a sock to a "cat's claw" (Figure 11-11). Request law enforcement personnel to conduct the search in your presence. If they refuse, complete a detailed survey of the patient and determine the number and extent of injuries before you accept the patient for transport.

When you are called to a scene and the patient is the suspected perpetrator of a violent crime, remove all of the patient's clothing while you conduct the survey and before you load the patient into the unit. This action will ensure that the patient is not armed. If this is not practical, immobilize the patient on a backboard to protect against spinal injury, which will also prevent the patient from reaching any concealed or makeshift weapons (Figure 11-12).

Do not allow women to carry a purse on the litter. The list of possible weapons that can be concealed in a purse is endless (Figure 11-13). Place the purse on the squad bench where it can be seen but not reached.

Figure 11-14 consists of photographs of makeshift or concealed weapons. Study them and determine how you would react to these items if you found them on a patient you were treating.

Text continued on p. 154.

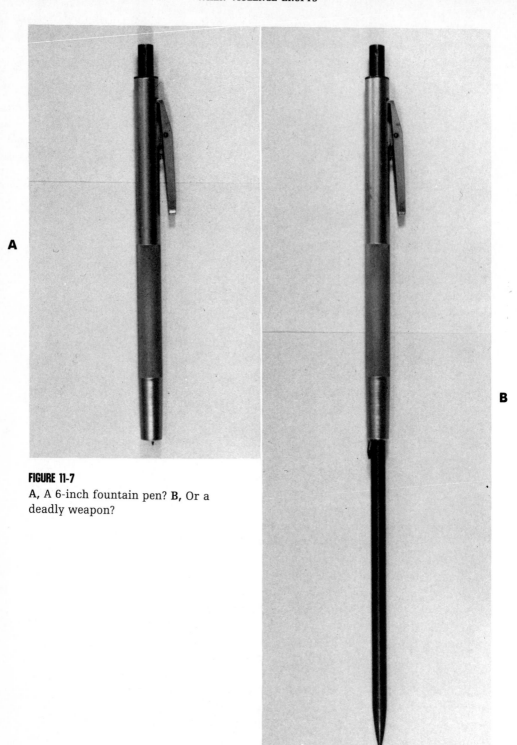

FIGURE 11-7
A, A 6-inch fountain pen? **B,** Or a
deadly weapon?

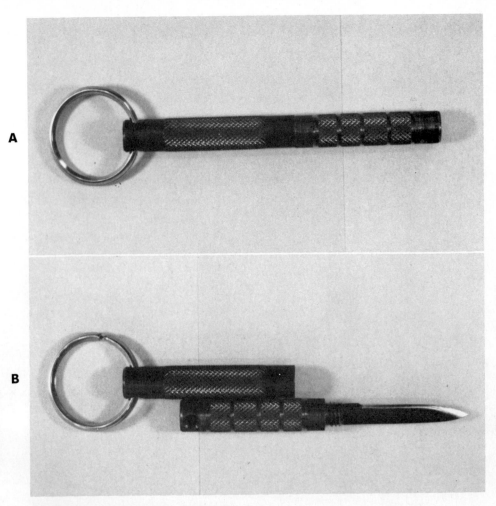

FIGURE 11-8
A, A harmless, 5-inch key ring? B, Or a deadly weapon?

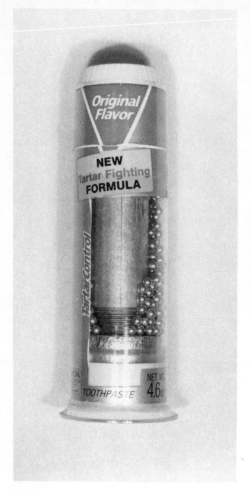

FIGURE 11-9
A toothpaste container with BBs that, when packed around a pipe bomb, become shrapnel when the device detonates.

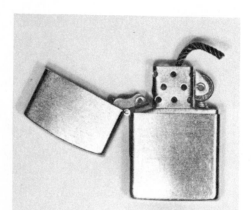

FIGURE 11-10
With the addition of explosives and a fuse, a lighter becomes an antipersonnel weapon.

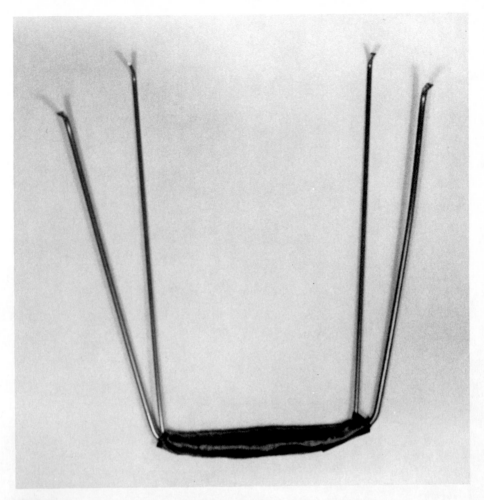

FIGURE 11-11
"Cat's claw" made from coat hangers with the tips shaved to a point. The weapon
is hand-held and raked across the victim's face.

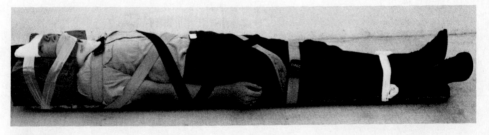

FIGURE 11-12
Shoestring strapping to hold patient on backboard to prevent spinal injury.

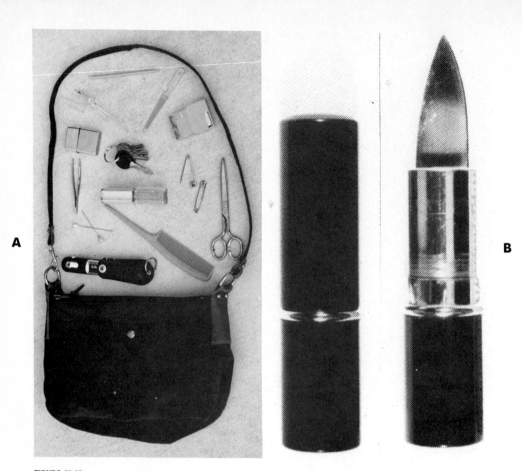

FIGURE 11-13

A, A women's purse can conceal an endless number of makeshift weapons. **B,** A lipstick tube conceals a knife.

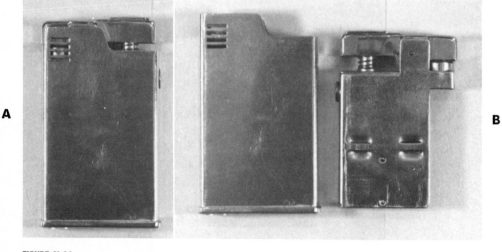

FIGURE 11-14

A, Cigarette lighter originally designed to fire small rounds of tear gas. **B,** It has been altered to fire a .22 caliber round.

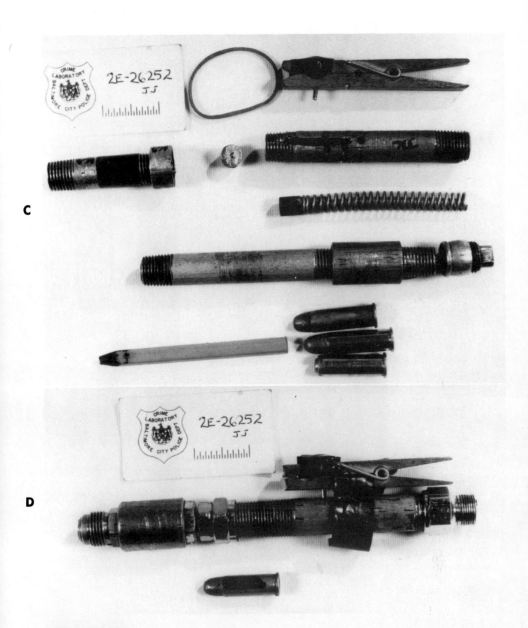

FIGURE 11-14, CONT'D.
C, Pipes, springs, clothespins, and rubber bands. D, Together they produce a
deadly weapon. *(Courtesy Baltimore City Police Department, Baltimore.)*

Continued.

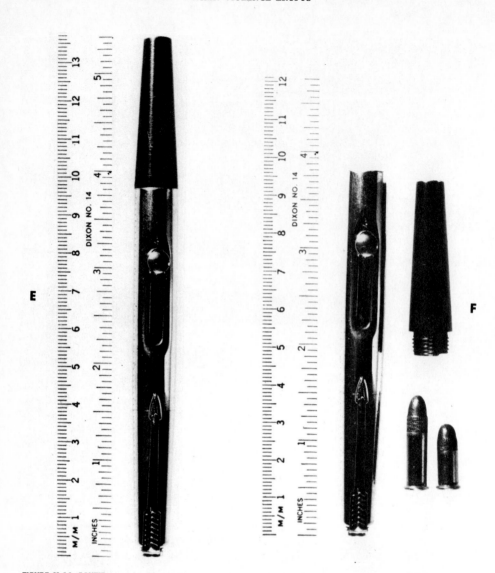

FIGURE 11-14, CONT'D.

E, Normal-looking pen. F, It fires a small-caliber round. *(Courtesy Baltimore City Police Department, Baltimore.)*

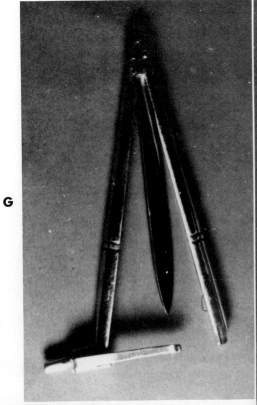

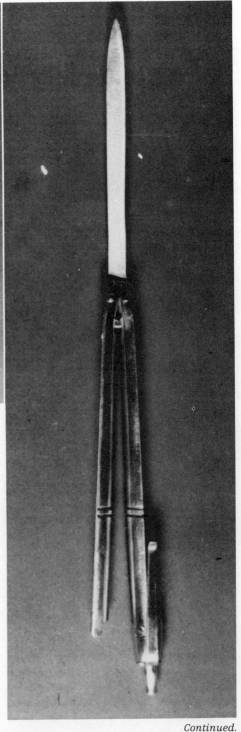

G

H

FIGURE 11-14, CONT'D.
G, Another normal-looking pen. **H,** It opens to form a knife. *(Courtesy Baltimore City Police Department, Baltimore.)*

Continued.

150

WHEN VIOLENCE ERUPTS

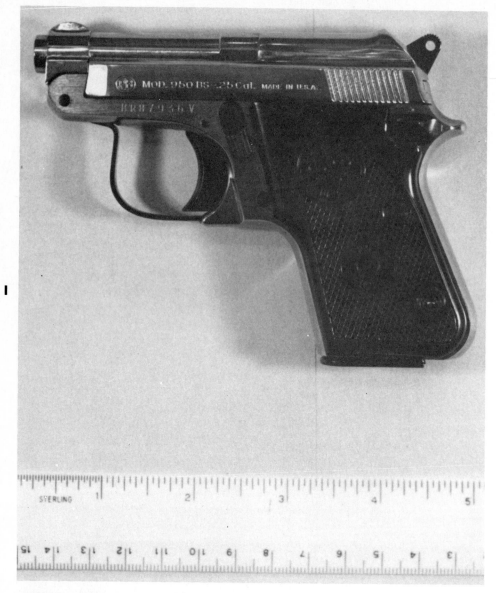

FIGURE 11-14, CONT'D.
I, A small-caliber, semiautomatic handgun that can be concealed in the palm of
the hand.

J

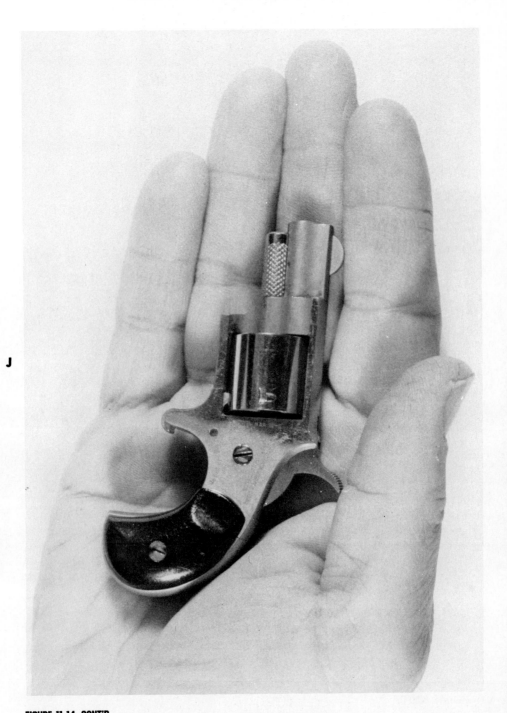

FIGURE 11-14, CONT'D.

J, A small-caliber revolver concealed in the palm of the hand. *(Courtesy Baltimore City Police Department, Baltimore.)*

Continued.

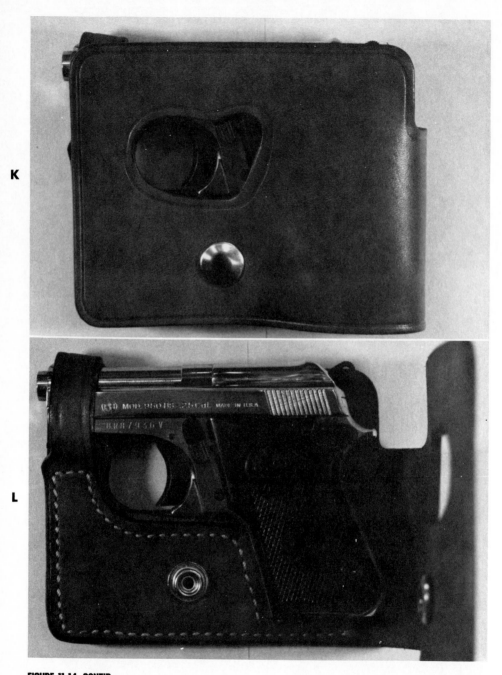

FIGURE 11-14, CONT'D.
K, A man's wallet. L, It contains a .25 caliber semiautomatic weapon. Pistol can be fired without opening the wallet.

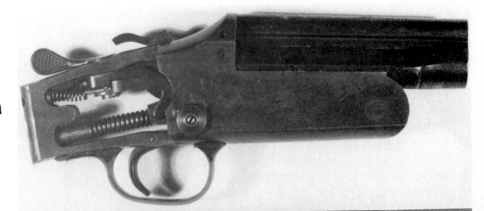

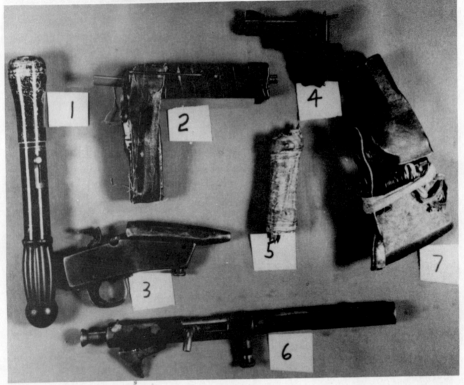

FIGURE 11-14, CONT'D.
M, An easily concealed shotgun with the stock and most of the barrel removed. **N,** Homemade guns of different calibers. *(Courtesy Baltimore City Police Department, Baltimore.)*

▼   **SURVIVAL TIPS**   ▼

1   A bomb that has not been located is a law enforcement problem—not yours.

2   An explosive device that has been located but not detonated is a law enforcement problem—not yours.

3   Booby traps have no memory. Once activated, anyone in the area is a potential victim, even the person who set the trap.

4   Never assume that a patient will not attack you because you are trying to help. Identify and move any items that can be used as makeshift weapons out of the patient's reach.

5   If you find an unusual object during your approach or patient care activities, withdraw to a safe area (taking the patient with you, if possible), and notify the proper authorities. Under no circumstances should anyone other than a trained bomb-disposal expert disturb the object.

6   If law enforcement personnel decide to inspect the object before calling the bomb squad, ask them to wait until you and your patient have moved a safe distance from the object.

7   Terrorists may set secondary explosive charges to disrupt a rescue operation.

8   It is better to have people laugh at you for being overcautious than to have them mourn you for being careless.

▼   ▼

12

CLANDESTINE DRUG LABORATORIES

The proliferation of illegal drug-manufacturing laboratories has increased the physical danger for emergency response personnel. Because of the efforts of law enforcement agencies in attempting to limit illegal drug trafficking from other countries, many drug merchants now make the products locally. The high demand for designer drugs has produced a lucrative market that encourages "do-it-yourself" experimentation. In December 1988 a Baltimore newspaper reported that chemicals purchased for $175 produce 1 pound of pure methamphetamine (speed or crank), which can be weakened and sold at a street value of $32,000.[1] Crank sales exceeded $3 billion in 1988, and production fell short of the 25-ton annual demand for the drug.[2]

Law enforcement raids on clandestine laboratories have more than tripled since 1983, with 775 labs shut down in 1987.[3] The problem is nationwide; the Western States Information Network reported 102 clandestine drug laboratories seized in Oregon in 1986.[4]

LOCATION OF ILLEGAL DRUG LABORATORIES

Clandestine drug laboratories are found in every geographic area. Socioeconomic conditions do not indicate possible locations of illegal drug labs. They can be found in cheap inner-city hotels, expensive homes in the suburbs, and small mobile homes throughout rural America. Labs are found in vehicles such as buses, trucks, and motor homes (Figure 12-1).

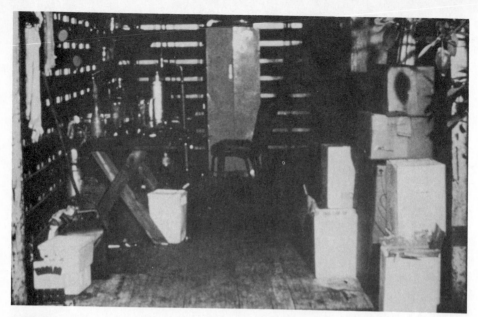

FIGURE 12-1
Rental vehicles may be used to transport chemicals to an illegal drug lab or are set up as a lab for cooking on the move. *(Courtesy Oregon State Fire Marshal's Office, Salem, Ore.)*

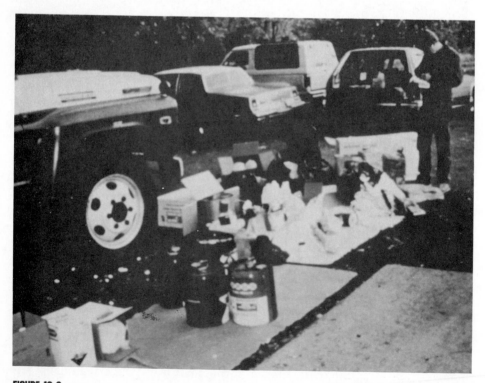

FIGURE 12-2
Police officer inventories chemicals and equipment removed from a mobile drug lab. *(Courtesy Oregon State Fire Marshal's Office, Salem, Ore.)*

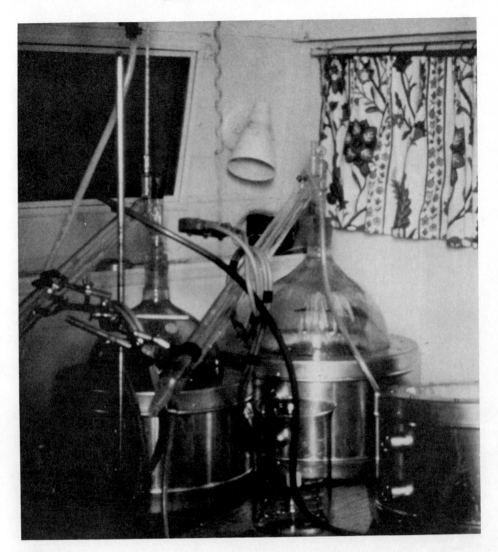

FIGURE 12-3
Clandestine drug lab with extensive glassware and sophisticated equipment.
(Courtesy Oregon State Fire Marshal's Office, Salem, Ore.)

The quality and quantity of equipment varies from the most basic laboratory that mixes compounds in buckets (Figure 12-2) to an elaborate laboratory that uses sophisticated glassware, heating mantles, and vacuum equipment (Figure 12-3).

RECOGNIZING ILLEGAL DRUG LABORATORIES

Fire and EMS personnel may be exposed to the dangers of an illegal drug lab if unsuspecting neighbors of a lab request the fire department to investigate unusual odors near their home. The odors produced during the

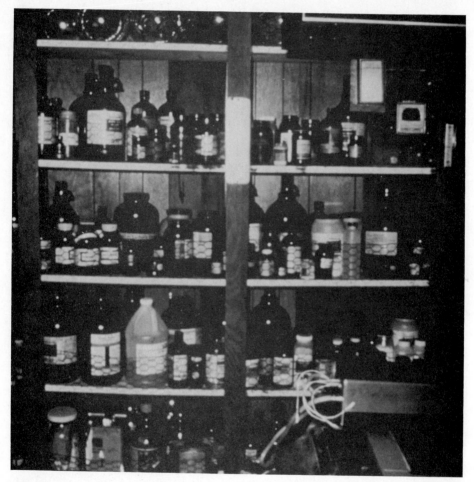

FIGURE 12-4
Chemical containers may not be properly labeled. *(Courtesy Oregon State Fire Marshal's Office, Salem, Ore.)*

cooking process in drug production can be mistaken for the smell of dried cat urine, cat litter, or rotten garbage. Many chemicals are used during the mixing process, including ether, which has a distinctive smell that many people recognize and report when calling for assistance (Figure 12-4).

Because of the highly flammable properties of many of the chemicals stored in an illegal drug lab, the response to a normal building or vehicle fire may turn into anything but a normal situation. After a dwelling fire that had been especially difficult to extinguish, firefighters in northern California discovered over 200 5-gallon drums of chemicals. The firefighters realized the house was being used as a clandestine drug lab and requested law enforcement assistance. Further investigation produced a large amount

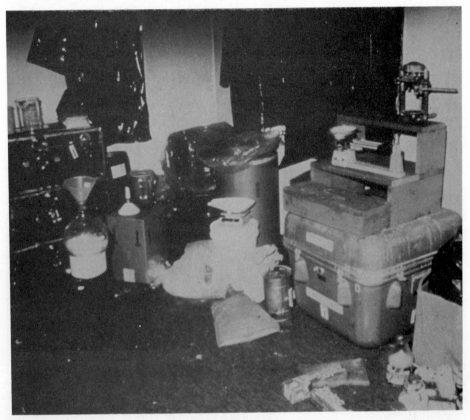

FIGURE 12-5
Crude equipment can produce most illegal drugs. *(Courtesy Oregon State Fire Marshal's Office, Salem, Ore.)*

of money, firearms and ammunition, and a cache of illegal drugs with a street value of $600,000. After inhaling toxic fumes, nine of the firefighters involved in the incident were taken to the hospital.[5]

Because many producers of illegal drugs use their own products, anticipate the possible discovery of an illegal drug lab whenever responding to a reported overdose. Watch for windows covered with black plastic, cardboard, or paint; they are often found at a structure containing an illegal drug lab. When you enter a building or vehicle to treat an overdose victim, look for glassware and other fundamental items that you might find in a high-school chemistry laboratory (Figure 12-5).

Persons working in illegal drug labs may request medical assistance if they develop symptoms of exposure to toxic, corrosive, explosive, or flammable materials. A list of chemicals that you may encounter is included in Appendix B.

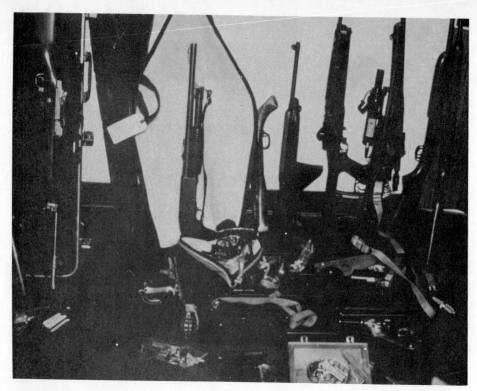

FIGURE 12-6
Booby traps, weapons, and explosives are found in illegal drug labs. *(Courtesy Oregon State Fire Marshal's Office, Salem, Ore.)*

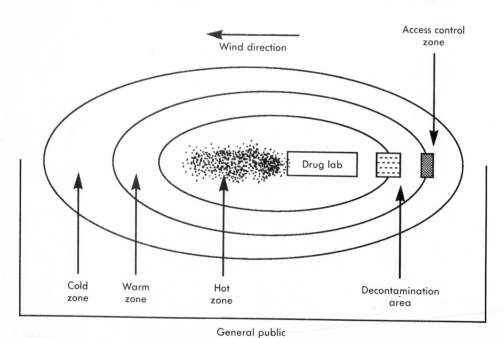

FIGURE 12-7
Establish safety zones for a hazardous-materials response.

HAZARDS ASSOCIATED WITH CLANDESTINE DRUG LABS

Every lab has a different configuration. You will not find a book of plans for constructing the perfect lab at your local bookstore. Recipes for drugs are usually handed down from one operator to another. *Everything* associated with a clandestine drug lab is hazardous! Be careful where you walk and avoid touching anything except the patient.

An action as simple as shutting off the tap-water supply to a cooling condenser can cause an explosion. Turning off the heat during a heat-induced chemical reaction is even more hazardous. Many chemical reactions must be shut down in stages, and only the operator understands the process used to shut down the system. Some cooking processes may require as long as 72 hours to complete. Because of the hazards of the cooking process, most operators will mix the ingredients and leave the area as soon as cooking begins.

To protect the operation, operators set booby traps. Outside mechanisms include fragmentation and incendiary devices, animal traps, and impaling stakes. Inside traps include vicious dogs, poisonous snakes, fishhooks hung at eye level, explosives connected to heating elements and electrical switches, and weapons such as crossbows and spear guns that discharge when the trigger mechanism is disturbed (Figure 12-6).

Contact explosives are the most common danger you will face while operating in an illegal drug lab.[6] These devices are made by combining potassium chlorate or red phosphorus with another chemical that becomes unstable when dried. The chemicals are rolled into a ball of aluminum foil and placed throughout the laboratory. If disturbed, the ball will explode.

Never disturb a suspected booby trap! Mark the location and notify the incident commander of the device. Do not use a portable radio to notify the incident commander; a radio transmission may activate an explosive device. Go to the command post and tell the commander in person.

EMERGENCY SCENE OPERATIONS

All personnel and equipment used at the scene of an illegal drug lab will be contaminated. After the area has been identified as a clandestine lab, establish a preliminary hazardous-materials *hot zone*. Include the lab and the area around the lab that contains all personnel and equipment in contact with the lab since the time of discovery (Figure 12-7). If equipment has been removed from the lab and placed on a vehicle, include the vehicle in the hot zone. When the hazardous-materials response team arrives on the scene, it will determine the boundaries of the zone.

After you are clear of the building or vehicle containing the lab, notify your dispatcher that you are at the scene of an illegal drug lab, and request that the following be notified to respond to the scene:

▶ Local law enforcement
▶ Drug Enforcement Administration

▸ Environmental Protection Agency
▸ Hazardous-materials response team
▸ Bomb squad
▸ Fire department for a full first-alarm response
▸ Additional EMS unit (ALS preferred)
▸ EMS supervisor
▸ Local health officials

EMS OPERATIONS

If an illegal drug lab is discovered during an emergency medical call, leave the lab immediately. Take the patient with you if you can without exposing yourself and your team to additional hazardous materials. If the patient is stable, remain in the preliminary hot zone until the hazardous-materials response team arrives on the scene. Unless you need specific equipment for patient treatment from your unit, do not return to it if it is outside the hot zone. You, your partner, your patient, and all equipment carried into the lab are considered contaminated until cleared by the hazardous-materials response team. Persons and equipment must be decontaminated before leaving the hot zone.

The hazardous-materials response team sets up and carries out decontamination procedures on *all* personnel and equipment leaving the hot zone. The decontamination stations are in a *warm zone,* which is contiguous to the hot zone. Access to the warm zone is limited to only those personnel directly involved in the incident.

If the condition of the patient requires immediate transport to a hospital, notify the medical facility of the circumstances. Explain that you have been exposed to unknown hazardous materials and that you and the patient have not been decontaminated. Request that the hazardous-materials response team respond to the hospital and carry out decontamination procedures there. Hospital personnel and equipment having contact with you, the patient, or your equipment must be included in the decontamination procedure (Figure 12-8).

FIRE SUPPRESSION OPERATIONS

When operating at a fire that is in or around a suspected drug lab, you must wear full protective clothing, including positive-pressure, self-contained breathing apparatus. Use higher levels of protective clothing, such as encapsulated suits, if chemicals are involved in the fire.

A hot zone must be established as soon as possible. Again, access to the hot zone is limited to personnel directly involved in fire suppression. Personnel from other agencies that will handle the chemicals, protect the environment, and collect evidence are not allowed past the warm zone until after the fire is out or the fire ground commander specifically authorizes their presence.

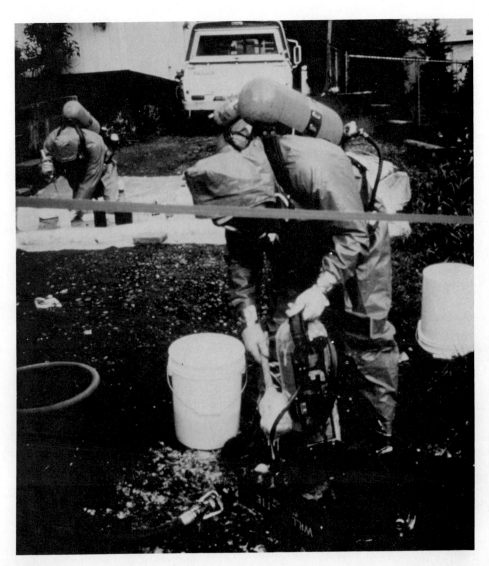

FIGURE 12-8
Proper protective clothing and complete decontamination must be part of standard
operating procedures for clandestine drug lab operations. *(Courtesy Oregon State
Fire Marshal's Office, Salem, Ore.)*

Identify the warm zone as soon as personnel can erect the decontamination stations. Backup personnel should move charged hose lines into the warm zone in anticipation of a rapid escalation of the fire. These personnel should be properly positioned, fully bunkered, and ready to advance into the hot zone.

The area within the boundary of the fire line or crime scene tape and outside of the warm zone should be established as a *cold zone*. This controlled area is off-limits to the general public. The incident command post is located in this area. Protective clothing is not required, and the area may be used to stage additional personnel and equipment.

If the structure or vehicle containing a known lab is burning when you arrive, protect the exposures and *let it burn*. Attempting to control the fire may prove deadly to the fire attack teams. Remember, the runoff of contaminated water produced by suppression efforts may cause widespread ecological damage.

If an initial fire attack is in progress when the location is identified as a drug lab, withdraw the attack teams and shift from offensive to defensive operations.

In all incidents involving drug labs, evacuate the structures on every side of the incident. When a fire or chemical spill is involved, consider evacuating people downwind from the incident.

POSITIVE-PRESSURE VENTILATION

Before you enter a known drug lab, remain outside and upwind from the location until the hazardous-materials response team ventilates the area and declares it safe. This should be the procedure for personnel responding to emergency medical situations, fire operations, chemical spills, and law enforcement activities.

Many of the chemicals used in clandestine drug labs are explosive if the proper air-to-product ratio is attained (see Appendix B). During the ventilation process this ratio will occur at some point, so all possible ignition sources must be eliminated to prevent an explosion during the ventilation process.

If mechanical ventilation of the structure or vehicle is required, use positive-pressure ventilation. All mechanical and power equipment remain outside of the area being ventilated, which further reduces the number of ignition sources during the ventilation process (Figure 12-9).

Check with the Drug Enforcement Administration's on-scene chemist before turning off any utilities. If the chemist has not arrived on the scene, wait before continuing the operation. After you receive permission from the chemist, secure all electric power from remote locations to prevent unwanted sparks or arcing (Figure 12-10).

To extinguish pilot lights on stoves, heaters, and furnaces, shut off all natural and low-pressure gas valves from outside the building. Do not shut off the gas if the on-scene chemist believes that it is not safe to remove the

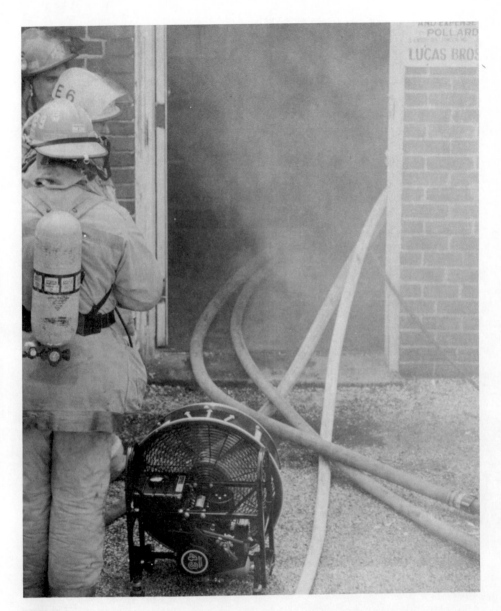

FIGURE 12-9

Positive-pressure ventilation is the only acceptable method of mechanical ventilation to use in drug lab operations. *(Courtesy Craig C. Schleunes, Baltimore County Fire Department, Baltimore.)*

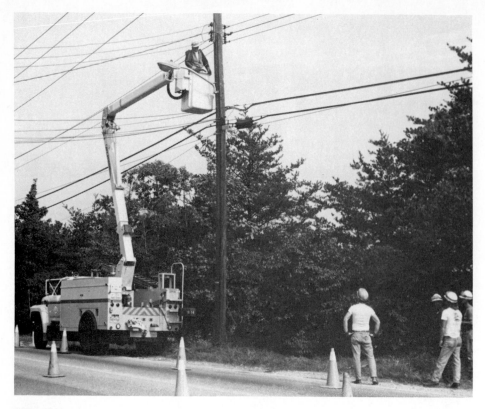

FIGURE 12-10
Trained personnel secure electric power to the suspected drug lab from a remote location.

heat from a chemical reaction already occurring. Withdrawing all personnel to the cold zone and waiting for the process to be complete may be necessary.

MONITORING PERSONNEL WORKING IN THE HOT ZONE

An ALS unit (BLS unit if ALS is not available) should be assigned to all clandestine drug lab operations to monitor *everyone* working in the hot zone. The unit establishes a monitoring station in the warm zone. All personnel leaving the hot zone report to the monitoring station for medical evaluation after decontamination.

Provide medical attention to anyone who develops any of the following symptoms associated with exposure to toxic chemicals:

▶ Nausea
▶ Vomiting
▶ Sharp headache

WARNING WARNING WARNING

A clandestine laboratory for the manufacture of illegal drugs and/or hazardous chemicals was seized at this location on _____ . Known hazardous chemicals have been disposed of pursuant to law.

However, there still may be hazardous substances or waste products on this property, either in buildings or in the ground itself. Please exercise caution while on these premises.

U.S. Department of Justice
Drug Enforcement Administration

Phone:

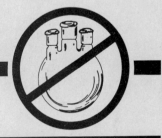

WARNING

FIGURE 12-11
Whenever you see this sign, treat the area as if the laboratory were still operating.

- ▶ Reddened face
- ▶ Burning sensation in the nose, throat, or lungs
- ▶ Drowsiness
- ▶ Numbness of lips
- ▶ Tingling teeth
- ▶ Eyes not focusing[7]

Chemicals used in labs can be absorbed into the walls and floors of the building. Although a lab was dismantled and all chemicals and equipment removed from the site days or even weeks earlier, a potential health hazard may still exist. The Drug Enforcement Administration posts warning signs on clandestine drug laboratories that have been seized and dismantled (Figure 12-11).

▼ SURVIVAL TIPS ▼

1 All personnel and agencies responding to an incident at an illegal drug lab need an immediate plan of action.
2 The time to plan for multiagency operations is not when a clandestine drug lab is discovered—it is *now!*
3 A drug lab is a crime scene—preserve the evidence!
4 Use only explosion-proof portable radios and flashlights in the hot zone.
5 Limit overhaul to extinguishing serious hot spots that may reignite or ignite residue vapors.

13

SELF-DEFENSE TACTICS

What should you do if the patient is being assaulted when you arrive? Should you jump in the middle of the fracas and protect the victim from harm? How would you react if an attack occurred while you or your crew were providing patient care?

When asked, prehospital care providers are likely to say, "Assist the assailant with oxygen therapy." The respondents are not talking about using a nasal cannula; they are talking about hitting the assailant on the head with a "D" cylinder. Although this technique is very effective, you and your department will probably face lawsuits.

How you use your voice is one of the most effective factors in controlling an incident (see Chapter 7). But if an aggressor ignores voice commands and continues to press forward, what action should you take? Should you use force against someone who is trying to hurt you or prevent you from reaching a patient?

REASONABLE USE OF FORCE

A *reasonable level of force* is the minimum amount of force needed to accomplish a goal. Emergency service providers must use a reasonable level of force to accomplish the following goals:

► Reach and treat any patient who is not breathing or has a blocked airway.

▶ Reach and treat any patient who is in cardiac arrest. The person could die if immediate corrective action is not taken.

▶ Reach and treat any patient with severe trauma.

▶ Remove any person interfering with patient care whenever the patient will die if the care is not continued.

▶ Move any person who attempts to prevent your retreat from a dangerous situation.

When you are faced with a situation that requires the use of force, always use a verbal challenge. Do not grab a person by the arm and pull. Physical contact with people is no longer acceptable conduct for emergency service workers as an initial line of defense.

If someone prevents you from reaching your patient, identify yourself and say, "Move back! That person may die if you don't let me help!" If the person blocking your way moves, you have attained your goal and no additional force is required. If the person does not move, take a side step and repeat the verbal challenge. Inform the person, "If you don't get out of my way, I'm calling the cops!" This threat usually makes the person move, but not always in the direction you wished. Be prepared to defend yourself.

Use physical force as a defensive technique, not an aggressive motion. Properly executed defensive motions can be as effective as physically striking your antagonist and are easier to defend if you face civil liability charges.

The amount of defensive force needed to protect yourself varies with each incident. If you feel that your life is in imminent danger, any action that will free you from the situation is a reasonable level of force.

THE INTERVIEW STANCE

If you are prepared, you can control an unexpected attack. Always use the interview stance so you will be in a defensive position if violence suddenly erupts. This stance is especially helpful in domestic encounters (see Chapter 9).

To assume the stance, stand approximately an arm's length from the person in front of you with your body at a 45-degree angle to the person. Have your feet a shoulder's width apart, your knees slightly bent, and your hands relaxed (Figure 13-1).

Look relaxed when you talk to the person. An unnatural stance signals that you are prepared for trouble and may cause the person to become aggressive (Figure 13-2).

If you practice, this stance will be automatic when you talk with a civilian. It is a comfortable way to stand and much safer than standing with your feet close together and facing the other person (Figure 13-3).

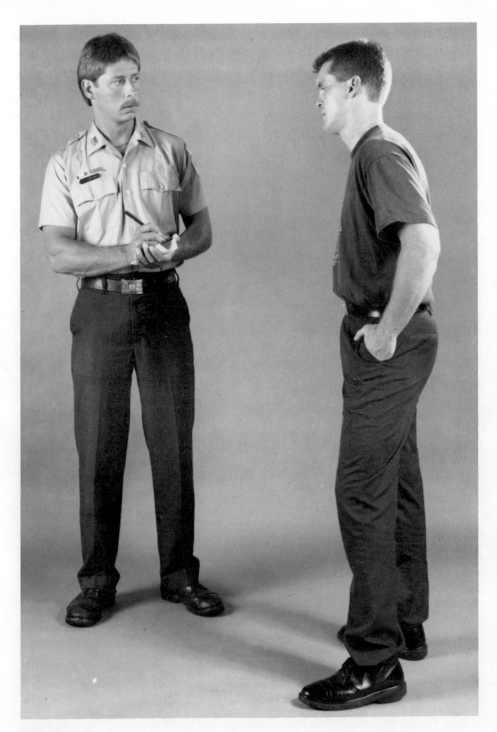

FIGURE 13-1
The interview stance.

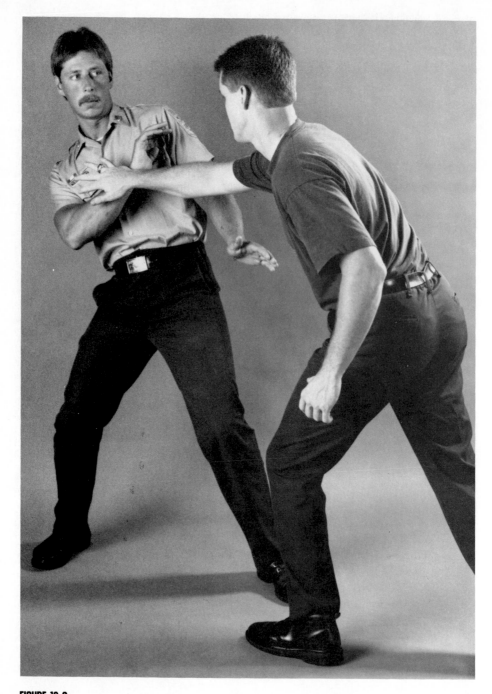

FIGURE 13-2

Using the interview stance facilitates balance and rapid movement to a more defensible position.

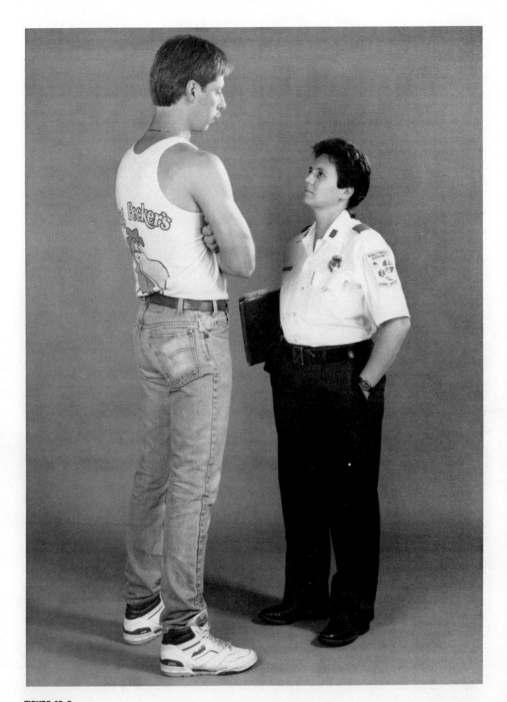

FIGURE 13-3
Do not stand with your feet together or your hands in your pockets when talking to a stranger.

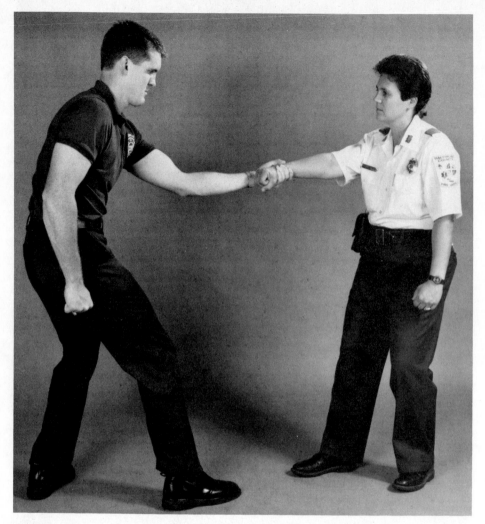

FIGURE 13-4
Normal reaction is to pull away.

THE WRIST GRASP

If someone unexpectedly grabs your wrist, your normal reaction is to pull away or jerk back from the attacker. Because you are controlled by the strength of the assailant's fingers, you will have difficulty in breaking the hold (Figure 13-4). If you jerk your forearm toward your body, you pull against the assailant's thumb (Figure 13-5) and can easily break the hold, since the thumb is much weaker than the combined strength of the fingers (Figure 13-6). Once the assailant's grip is released, retreat to a safe area.

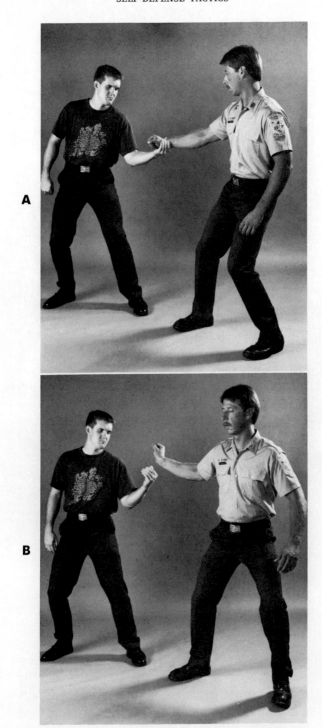

FIGURE 13-5
A, Pull toward the thumb. B, Break the hold, and turn and run.

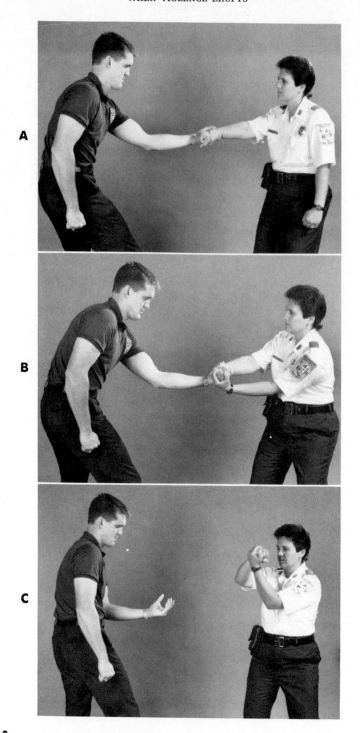

FIGURE 13-6

A, The attacker's grip is too strong for you to pull free when pulling against the thumb. B, Use your free hand to increase pulling power. C, Reach between you and your assailant, grab your trapped hand, and pull yourself free.

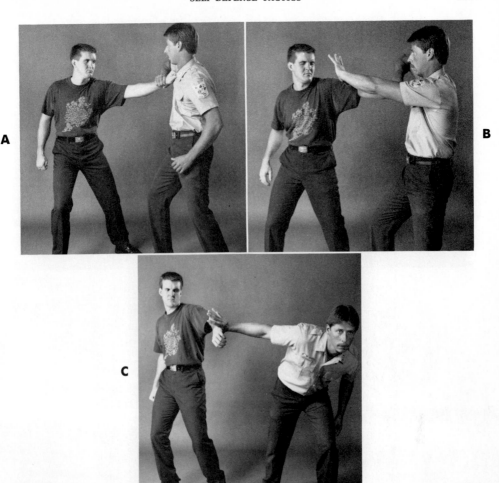

FIGURE 13-7
A, Seize your attacker's hand and twist toward the thumb. B, Move your free hand toward your attacker's face, which will break the concentration long enough for you to escape. C, After you feel the grip relaxing on your shirt, twist your body away from your assailant and run to a safer area.

TECHNIQUE FOR DISTRACTING AN ASSAILANT

If an assailant grabs the front of your shirt, seize the hand of the attacker and twist toward the thumb. At the same time, flash your free hand through the assailant's field of vision. This unexpected action should break the person's concentration long enough for you to break the hold and escape (Figure 13-7).

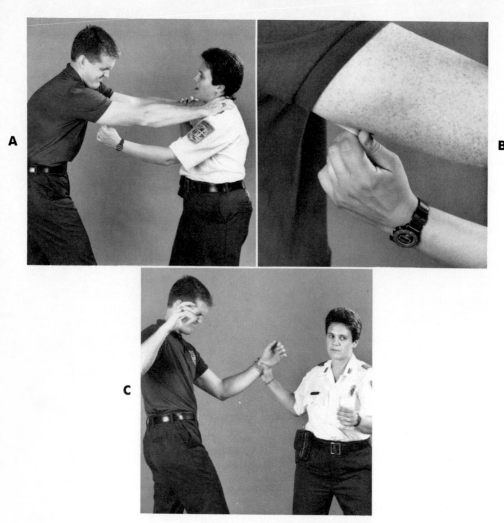

FIGURE 13-8

A, One way to break a front stranglehold is to apply a tweak. **B,** Pinch, pull, and twist a small piece of skin under the arm. **C,** As soon as you feel the assailant's grip relax, twist and run.

THE POWER OF A TWEAK

A *tweak* is performed by pinching a small piece of skin under a person's upper arm. If you pinch, twist, and pull at the same time, you can bring most people to their knees, regardless of size. This move is most painful when applied directly to the skin (Figure 13-8). If the assailant is wearing a long-sleeved shirt or jacket, a tweak may not be effective.

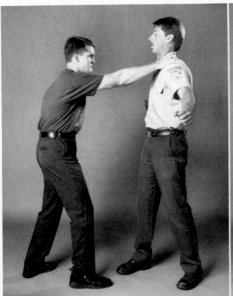

A

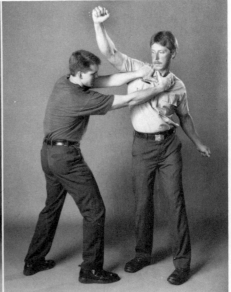

B

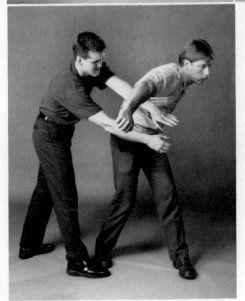

C

FIGURE 13-9
A, The moment someone you are facing attempts to strangle you, extend both arms. B, Rotate either arm in a windmill motion to break the hold. C, As soon as the hold is broken, *run!*

BREAKING A STRANGLEHOLD WHEN ATTACKED FROM THE FRONT

If an assailant tries to strangle you from the front, raise both arms outward from the sides of your body. Rotate either arm in a windmill motion, using your upper arm to hit the assailant's wrist and break the hold. Do this movement quickly and with as much physical force as possible (Figure 13-9).

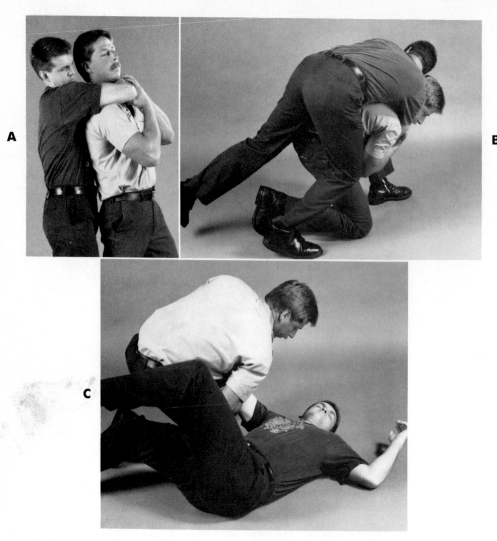

FIGURE 13-10
A, If attacked from the right, grab your assailant's right forearm and pull toward your chest. **B,** At the same time drop to your right knee, and turn your body toward the assailant. **C,** Once the hold is broken, get up and *run!*

BREAKING A STRANGLEHOLD APPLIED FROM THE REAR

If your assailant places a right arm around your neck, use both of your hands to pull the assailant's forearm toward your chest. At the same time, drop to your right knee and twist your body to the left. Your assailant will lose balance and be thrown to the ground directly in front of you. As soon as the hold is broken, get up and run (Figure 13-10).

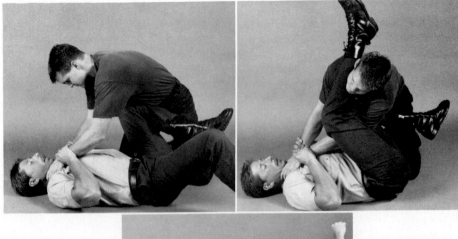

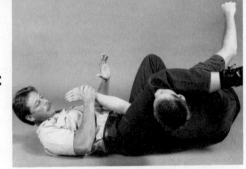

FIGURE 13-11

A, To break a stranglehold from above, bring your right knee up against the assailant's hip or stomach and grab both of the assailant's wrists. **B,** Swing your left leg up, hook it under the assailant's chin, and push toward the ground. **C,** Your assailant loses the grip on your throat and falls backward to the ground. You can now escape to a safer area.

If your assailant places a left arm around your neck, drop to your left knee while pulling the assailant's left forearm toward your chest and twisting your body to the right. The result will be the same. The assailant will be thrown off-balance and land on the ground in front of you.

BREAKING A STRANGLEHOLD APPLIED FROM ABOVE

Patients are often found on the floor or ground or are placed there by emergency response personnel. To provide patient care at this level, you must kneel or squat next to the patient. In either position, you are very vulnerable to an unexpected attack from above. An assailant can easily gain a stranglehold and wrestle you to the ground.

In Figure 13-11, an assailant is strangling a paramedic after attacking him from the right. The paramedic uses the leg-bar technique to break free.

PRACTICE

The self-defense tactics presented in this chapter can save your life if properly applied. The only way you will learn to apply these techniques is to practice each one under controlled conditions. You must practice until you can do every motion without thinking. A qualified instructor should supervise practice sessions until the technique is mastered.

After a technique is mastered, continue to practice so that you can maintain the skill level needed to apply the technique quickly and correctly. An automatic response can be developed only through practice. Your reaction to attack must be automatic; there is no time to think when violence erupts.

DOCUMENTATION

Report any threatened or actual assaults to the police. Even though the incident may have seemed insignificant, file a police report.

If you are required to defend yourself and use one of the techniques presented in this chapter, state the facts clearly and completely in the police report. Anytime you put your hands on someone during the course of your duties for reasons other than providing patient care, ensure that the reasons are documented, placed on file, and available for use in case of litigation.

▼   SURVIVAL TIPS   ▼

1 You do not have the authority, training, or responsibility to subdue a person who is preventing you from reaching your patient. That is the police department's responsibility.
2 If your professional knowledge warns you that a person will die if not helped immediately, verbally force your way to the victim. If you fail to reach the patient, call for police assistance, be *extremely forceful* in your verbal demands, and be ready to defend yourself.
3 Know the local laws about fire and EMS personnel using force.
4 Never carry or use an unauthorized weapon to defend yourself or your patient.
5 Remember, you can be sued for any action you take. Individual departments must formulate written policy to protect personnel if they are involved in a physical confrontation during the course of their duties.
6 When you use the self-defense techniques presented in this chapter, use them with all the physical strength you possess. You are fighting for your life.

14

SWAT MEDICS

Because you are a member of a fire, rescue or EMS emergency response team, you can expect to be called to riot scenes, areas where suspected criminals are barricaded, hostage situations, and other potentially explosive incidents. All of these situations are law enforcement problems and are usually handled by a law enforcement agency. The police operate inside a clearly identified police zone, and fire suppression and EMS personnel wait outside in a staging area unless needed.

If a situation suddenly deteriorates and someone is injured or the police need special assistance from the fire suppression personnel, you may be called from the controlled staging area and asked to enter a potentially dangerous police zone. Most fire, rescue, and EMS personnel thrust into this situation are not trained to operate under these conditions, have no interest in receiving the training, and should not be expected to perform such duties.

Many local governments, recognizing the need for specially trained personnel to handle violent incidents, have assembled special weapons and tactics (SWAT) teams from local law enforcement agencies. SWAT teams consist of highly motivated, highly trained, and sincerely dedicated police officers who are individually selected from a list of qualified volunteers (Figure 14-1).

Agencies recognize the need to have competent medical care available at the scene of any incident involving SWAT intervention. The volatile atmosphere surrounding SWAT team operations is conducive to severe injury to the individuals at the location and requires the immediate availabil-

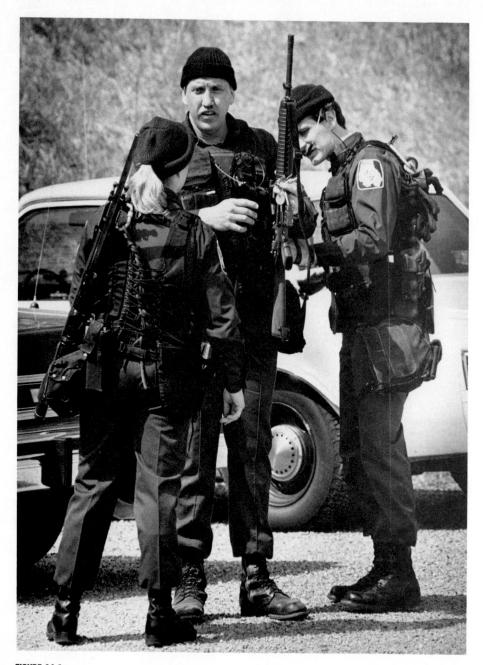

FIGURE 14-1
Members of the Baltimore County SWAT team check their gear before taking their positions during a hostage situation. *(Courtesy Charles Weiss, Columbia, Md, Patuxent Publishing Company.)*

ity of advanced life-support services. To meet this need, some jurisdictions assign selected fire, rescue, and EMS personnel to law enforcement agencies to train and work with SWAT teams. Personnel selected to participate in this program are called SWAT medics.

Any operation involving a SWAT team and SWAT medics requires a large number of support personnel from all agencies. Police, fire, rescue, and EMS personnel assigned to the incident who are not trained SWAT team members *must* remain outside of the SWAT team's operating perimeter.

THE TEAM

No national standards for recognition as a SWAT medic exist, and team size varies depending on local needs. Whenever fire, rescue, and EMS personnel are assigned to a SWAT team, they must operate in pairs, not independently from other medical personnel. In Bellingham, Washington,[1] and Miami, Florida,[2] paramedic certification is a prerequisite to participation in the SWAT medic program.

All SWAT medics must have an intimate knowledge of all SWAT team operating procedures. SWAT medics must understand the reaction of criminals to SWAT team activities so that they can determine the necessary procedures for effective patient care. In some situations a patient cannot be moved until the hostile environment is stabilized. The SWAT medic must be emotionally and professionally prepared to provide quality patient care while surrounded by a hostile environment.

SWAT medics, as well as all SWAT team members, spend countless off-duty hours engaged in physical conditioning. In addition to the usual fire, rescue, EMS, or law enforcement duties, they must also develop and maintain advanced hand-to-hand combat skills and be highly proficient in the use of all equipment and medical supplies that are part of the standard issue (Figure 14-2).

When SWAT medics need to learn special-weapons skills, they are under strict control in their handling of weapons. Although Rapides Parish in Alexandria, Louisiana, commissions Emergency Medical Tactical Response (EMTAC) team members as "Special Medical Deputies"[3] and Miami commissions team members as "Special Officers,"[4] SWAT medics are not considered an aggressive part of an assault team. Their presence is for immediate advanced life-support services in a hostile area. Weapons assigned to SWAT medic personnel are used only in self-defense.

TRAINING

The intensity of emergency medical training and the amount of police training required for fire, rescue, and EMS personnel to qualify as SWAT medics are determined by the authority having jurisdiction over the SWAT

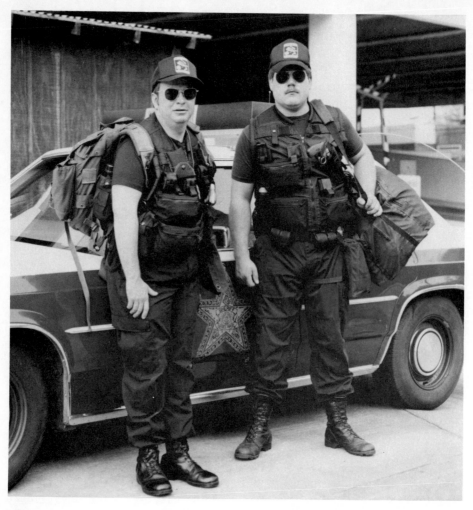

FIGURE 14-2
SWAT medics dressed for work. *(Courtesy Kathy Calongne, Pineville, La.)*

team. The Miami program requires 40 hours of police training; Rapides Parish requires almost 140 hours. You will find an outline of the Rapides Parish training program in Appendix C.

Weapon's training ranges from the use of a handgun to the MAC-10 machine gun. Medics study and practice basic SWAT team techniques and search procedures. Medics receive extensive training in specific skills, depending on local conditions. For example, teams operating in metropolitan areas devote many hours to rappelling from helicopters and buildings and spend little time on the techniques of land navigation, while teams in rural areas may have the opposite training priorities.

SWAT medics are taught about hostage negotiations, not to be qualified as hostage negotiators but to be familiarized with the dynamics of the

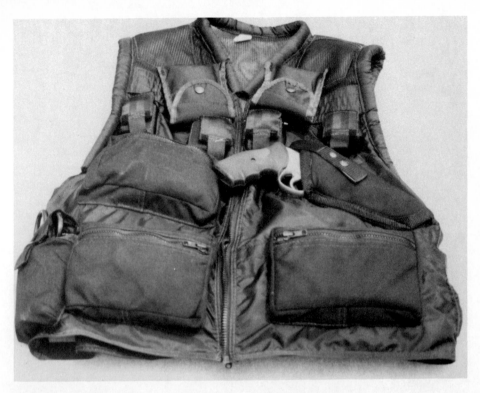

FIGURE 14-3
Load-bearing vests hold the contents of an aid bag, assorted personal equipment, and a weapon. *(Courtesy Rapides Parish Sheriff's Department, Alexandria, La.)*

process. Some operations may last for several days. If SWAT medics understand the overall plan of the police officers assigned to the SWAT team, they will not experience impatience or boredom during a hostage situation.

The intent of SWAT medic training is not to certify fire, rescue, or emergency medical personnel as police officers, but to teach them to think and act as police officers when participating in extremely dangerous operations. In many areas, members of the local police department SWAT team train personnel from the other emergency services; the training is also available from the FBI.

EQUIPMENT

Fire, rescue, and emergency medical personnel assigned to SWAT teams are usually issued fatigue uniforms similar to those worn by law enforcement members of the team. Firearms may be issued for the duration of the incident and only for defensive purposes.[5]

Because SWAT medics must be mobile, they carry only the equipment that is considered absolutely necessary (Figure 14-3). Backpacks and load-bearing vests carry vital-signs monitoring equipment, intravenous (IV) so-

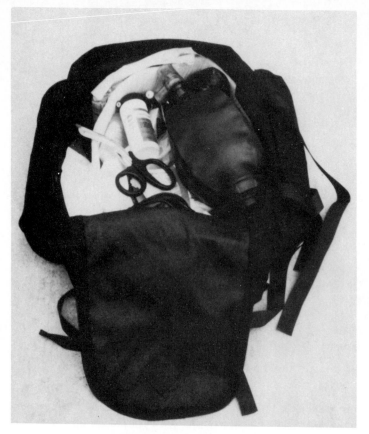

FIGURE 14-4
EMTAC individual medical bag. *(Courtesy Rapides Parish Sheriff's Department, Alexandria, La.)*

lutions, and carefully selected medical supplies. ALS kits contain only those items needed for major trauma injuries. MAST trousers should be standard equipment for all SWAT medic teams. Morphine sulfate must be available to the team, but local protocols will dictate how this is accomplished.

A list of individual equipment (Figure 14-4) and medical equipment (Figure 14-5) carried by the Rapides Parish EMTAC team is found in Appendix D.

RESPONSIBILITIES OF A SWAT MEDIC

The first responsibility of a SWAT medic is to move an injured person to temporary cover and begin appropriate patient care. Surrounding circumstances and current operating conditions affect your ability to accomplish this goal.

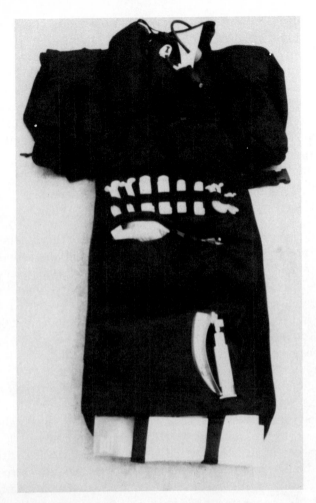

FIGURE 14-5
EMTAC team medical bag. *(Courtesy Rapides Parish Sheriff's Department, Alexandria, La.)*

During the initial stage of patient treatment, rely on standing orders issued by the local medical director responsible for patient care. Standing orders must allow you to perform advanced life-support operations (including IV therapy, airway management, and MAST therapy) without communicating with the team leader or medical director. The extent of patient care you can provide at this time is limited by the amount and type of equipment you can carry into the forward operating area.

Move your patient to a designated, secure collecting point outside of the kill zone and within the perimeter of police operations as soon as possible. The collecting point should be protected by SWAT team personnel until the incident has ended.

The team leader (located in the command post) is responsible for assembling additional equipment at the collecting point. You will need a team ALS kit, a cardioscope, and backboards to continue patient stabilization and advanced life-support procedures. Because most of this equipment is too cumbersome to carry on your person, remove it from standby medic units in the staging area. Package the stabilized patient for transport and move under SWAT team protection to the police zone perimeter. Transfer the patient to a medic crew for transport to a medical facility. Medical units or fire apparatus must never be within the police zone perimeter until the area is secured.

▼   SURVIVAL TIPS   ▼

1   Know the objectives of a SWAT medic program—they are as important to your safety as any survival tip in this book. The dependency between law enforcement personnel and other emergency responders is emphasized more in SWAT medic/SWAT team operations than in any other emergency you will encounter.

2   If you are not training or working as an active member of a SWAT medic team, *do not* enter the operating perimeter. Until the SWAT team has secured the area and your agency is authorized to take over, remain in the staging area.

3   SWAT medic operations are usually conducted in a hostile environment, and medical communications may not be possible. Consult your medical director and obtain a written set of standing orders that includes airway management, IV therapy, and MAST therapy procedures.

4   A SWAT medic team leader responds to all emergencies with the team. The team leader reports to the command post, assumes responsibility for all medical activities, maintains contact with team members operating within the perimeter, and, most importantly, acts as a liaison between the host law enforcement agency and the fire, rescue, and EMS personnel.

▼   ▼

APPENDIX A

SOFT BODY ARMOR

Concern for the safety of emergency service personnel in the United States is increasing. The weapons used on the street today have changed drastically from those used several years ago. In the past, street people used "Saturday night specials," little, small-caliber handguns, often held together by bailing wire or tape. Today these people are armed with sophisticated weapons ranging from small, 9 mm pistols to compact automatic-assault weapons. Because of the growing use of these deadly weapons, fire protection agencies, individual firefighters, and EMS personnel are realizing the importance of using soft body armor.

In Houston, Texas, ambulances are equipped with soft body armor for firefighter paramedics.[1] Approximately 12 of the 364 EMS personnel in the City of Los Angeles Fire Department voluntarily wear soft body armor full-time. The department also provides, on an optional basis, body armor protection to all personnel who will be involved in specific assignments.[2]

Catalogs advertising collectibles, uniforms, books, and training materials mailed to fire service personnel now include advertisements for soft body armor.[3] Publishers of law enforcement periodicals, which have featured soft body armor ads for years, are now including fire and EMS professionals on their unsolicited mailing lists.[4]

Violence toward fire, rescue, and EMS personnel continues to escalate. Individuals, as well as entire departments, will probably purchase soft body armor in the future. Knowing its construction and protection qualities will help you to decide what type of equipment to purchase.

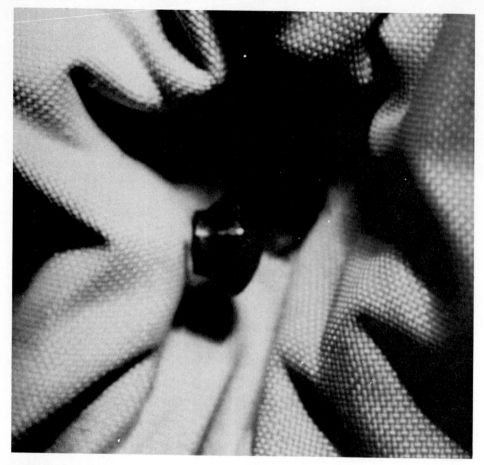

FIGURE A-1

Bullet bouncing off soft body armour. *(Courtesy E.I. Du Pont De Nemours and Company, Wilmington, Del.)*

Contrary to popular belief, Kevlar is not bulletproof, but it is recognized as the preferred material for bullet- and fragment-resistant protective apparel.[5] It was introduced in 1972 by E.I. Du Pont De Nemours and Company. Since that time, it has been blended with natural cloth and synthetic material to produce work uniforms and protective clothing for emergency service workers. An ounce of Kevlar is 5 times stronger than an equal weight of steel, extremely stretch-resistant, inherently flame-resistant, and will not melt.[6]

A bullet striking any object produces energy. When a bullet strikes a Kevlar vest, the fibers surrounding the point of impact absorb and dissipate the initial shock of the bullet over a large area, thus preventing the projectile from penetrating the material and reducing the possibility of blunt trauma (Figure A-1). Bruises, lacerations, and some internal injuries

THREAT LEVEL CHART

THREAT LEVEL	BALLISTIC PROTECTION
I	.22 caliber long rifle handgun rounds .38 caliber special projectiles
IIA	.22 caliber long rifle handgun rounds .38 caliber special projectiles .357 Magnum 158 grain striking at 1250 ft/sec 9 mm 124 grain striking at 1090 ft/sec
II	.22 caliber long rifle handgun rounds .38 caliber special projectiles .357 Magnum 158 grain striking at 1250 ft/sec .357 Magnum 158 grain striking at 1395 ft/sec 9 mm 124 grain striking at 1090 ft/sec 9 mm 124 grain striking at 1175 ft/sec
IIIA	.22 caliber long rifle handgun rounds .38 caliber special projectiles .357 Magnum 158 grain striking at 1250 ft/sec .357 Magnum 158 grain striking at 1395 ft/sec 9 mm 124 grain striking at 1090 ft/sec 9 mm 124 grain striking at 1175 ft/sec .977 124 grain striking at 1400 ft/sec .44 Magnum semi wad cutter striking at 1400 ft/sec
III	.22 caliber long rifle handgun rounds .38 caliber special projectiles .357 Magnum 158 grain striking at 1250 ft/sec .357 Magnum 158 grain striking at 1395 ft/sec 9 mm 124 grain striking at 1090 ft/sec 9 mm 124 grain striking at 1175 ft/sec .977 124 grain striking at 1400 ft/sec .44 Magnum semi wad cutter striking at 1400 ft/sec 7.62 mm (308 Winchester)
IV	.22 caliber long rifle handgun rounds .38 caliber special projectiles .357 Magnum 158 grain striking at 1250 ft/sec .357 Magnum 158 grain striking at 1395 ft/sec 9 mm 124 grain striking at 1090 ft/sec 9 mm 124 grain striking at 1175 ft/sec .977 124 grain striking at 1400 ft/sec .44 Magnum semi wad cutter striking at 1400 ft/sec 7.62 mm (308 Winchester) 30.06 projectiles

may occur if you are struck by a bullet or fragments while wearing soft body armor. If you are shot while wearing soft body armor, you must be examined at a medical facility.

Not all body armor is equally strong. It is classified into six levels of protection. The threat level chart shown in the box is offered only as a guideline. Before you purchase any soft body armor, you must know the type of weapons being used on the street.[7] Keep abreast of this changing information and adjust your level of protection accordingly. In all instances, make sure the body armor you have purchased meets or exceeds the specifications required by the current National Institute of Justice Standard No. 0101.03.

Adjusting to the feel of wearing body armor takes time. New vests may feel bulky until you become accustomed to this feeling. During summer months, expect to feel hot and somewhat uncomfortable. Remember that the vest is giving you added protection, and any discomfort you may experience is a small price to pay for this protection.

Specific instructions for the care of your body armor are provided by the manufacturer; however, the following guidelines apply to all brands:

- Hand wash the body armor in cold water with a mild detergent.
- Thoroughly rinse and remove *all* detergent. (An improperly rinsed vest can develop reduced stopping power.)
- Never use bleach or any product containing bleach.
- Never dry clean. (Check manufacturer's specifications.)
- Never machine wash or machine dry.
- Always drip-dry indoors.
- Return the vest to the manufacturer for repairs.[8]

Inspect your body armor regularly. Look for signs of abrasion, fabric fraying, or unravelling. A washed-out appearance or permanent wrinkles indicate unusual wear. Ensure that the vest fits properly and is relatively comfortable. Armor should be replaced after it has stopped a bullet or after 5 years of normal use. Do not abuse the vest; treat it as if your life depends on it—*it does.*

▼   ▼

APPENDIX B

CHEMICALS USED IN CLANDESTINE DRUG LABS

You must exercise extreme caution when operating at the scene of an illegal drug lab. Do not walk into, touch, or move chemicals or spilled material. Avoid inhaling fumes, smoke, and vapors, even if it is not known if chemicals are involved. Never assume that gases or vapors are harmless because they do not have an odor.

Table B-1, pp. 197-201, is similar to a table found in the Oregon State Fire Marshal's *Student Manual for Hazardous Materials Technician I Certification.* Additional information on chemicals associated with drug lab operations was taken from the Sacramento Fire Department's *Hazardous Material Response Team Operations and Policies.*

Any of the listed chemicals may be found in or around a clandestine drug lab. Many are explosive, toxic, and/or flammable. All details of the listed chemicals are not known, and all chemicals that may be found on a scene are not contained in the list. Assume any chemical found in a drug lab is hazardous.

The following resources and definitions will assist you in identifying the dangers of chemicals in an illegal drug lab:

- ► U.S. Department of Transportation (DOT) Emergency Response Guidebook (ERG) Number: If you know the name of the product, look in the alphabetical index for the ERG number. Turn to the numbered guide page, read carefully, and proceed as recommended.
- ► United Nations (UN) Identification Number: If you do not know the name of the product, use the UN number as a cross-reference in the

Emergency Response Guidebook to the ERG number. Again, turn to the numbered guide page, read carefully, and proceed as recommended.

▸ Hazard Identification: The hazard identification number is based on the National Fire Protection Association's (NFPA) 704, *Standard System for the Identification of the Fire Hazards of Materials* (1985). Material hazards are rated according to the three categories of health, flammability, and reactivity. The severity of danger for each category ranges from 0 (no danger) to 4 (severe hazard).

▸ Explosive, Poisonous, Corrosive: If a chemical is labeled with one of these terms, turn to the numbered guide page of the chemical in the ERG, read carefully, and proceed as recommended.

▸ Precursor: A substance that is the source of another substance. Precursors are used to create chemical compounds that cannot be obtained legitimately.

▸ Solvent: A substance that dissolves another substance. Solvents "wash" chemical compounds produced during the stages of the conversion process.

▸ Reagent: A substance used in a chemical reaction.

Every emergency vehicle should have a current edition of the *Emergency Response Guidebook.* The information in this book can save your life, not only during an incident at a drug lab, but at any incident involving chemicals and other hazardous materials.

If your organization has not received free copies of the ERG from your state or local distribution center, call the Hazardous Materials Information Exchange to obtain the telephone number of your state coordinator. The toll free number for the exchange is 1-800-752-6367. In Illinois, call 1-800-367-9562.

TABLE B-1

Chemicals used in clandestine drug labs

Chemical	UN number	ERG number	Health hazard rating	Flammability hazard rating	Reactivity hazard rating	Explosive	Poisonous	Corrosive	Precursor	Solvent	Reagent	Comments
Acetaldehyde (Ethanal)	1089	26	2	4	2	*	*	*	*			
Acetic acid	1842	29	2	2	1	*	*	*		*		
Acetic acid ethyl ester (Ethyl acetate)	1173	26	1	3	0	*	*			*		
Acetic anhydride	1715	39	2	2	1	*	*	*	*			Avoid water, caustics, and alcohol.
Acetonitrile (Ethanenitrile)	1648	28	2	3	0	*	*	*	*			
Aluminum chloride, anhydrous	1726	39	3	0	2		*	*			*	Avoid water; rubber overclothing required.
Ammonia, anhydrous	1005	15	2	1	0		*	*	*			
Ammonium acetate	9079	31	–	–	–				*	*		Produces poison gas while burning.
Ammonium chloride	9085	31	2	0	0				*	*		Produces poison gas while burning.
Ammonium hydroxide (Household ammonia)	2672	60	–	–	–		*	*	*			
Anhydrous hydriodic acid (Hydrogen iodide)	2197	15	3	0	0		*	*			*	
Benzene	1114	27	2	3	0	*	*	*	*			Suspected carcinogen.
Benzeneacetonitrile (Benzyl cyanide)	–	–	–	–	–	*	*	*	*			Suspected carcinogen.
Benzenesulfonyl chloride	2225	59	–	–	–		*				*	Suspected carcinogen.
Boron trifluoride	1008	15	3	0	1		*	*			*	
Bromobenzene	2514	26	–	–	–	*	*				*	Suspected carcinogen.
2-Butanone (Methyl ethyl ketone)	1193	26	1	3	0	*	*	*	*			

Dashed entries (—) = information not available.
Modified from Oregon State Fire Marshal's Training Bureau.

Continued.

TABLE B-1

Chemicals used in clandestine drug labs—cont'd

Chemical	UN number	ERG number	Health hazard rating	Flammability hazard rating	Reactivity hazard rating	Explosive	Poisonous	Corrosive	Precursor	Solvent	Reagent	Comments
Calcium hydroxide (Slaked lime)	–	–	–	–	–						*	
(Chloromethyl)benzene (Benzyl chloride)	1738	59	2	2	1		*				*	Suspected carcinogen.
1-Chloro-2-propanone (Chloroacetone)	1695	56	–	–	–	*	*	*	*			
Copper sulfate	–	–	–	–	–						*	
Cyclohexanone	1915	26	1	2	0	*	*	*			*	
N,N-Diethylethanamine (Triethylamine)	1296	68	2	3	0		*	*			*	Produces poison gas while burning; rubber overclothing required.
N,N-Dimethylformamide	2265	26	1	2	0	*	*	*				Essential for drug production.
Ethanamine (Ethylamine)	1036	68	3	4	0	*	*				*	
Ethanedioic acid (Oxalic acid)	–	–	2	1	0		*	*			*	Rubber overclothing required.
Ethanol (Ethyl alcohol)	1170	26	0	3	0	*	*	*		*		
Formaldehyde solution (Formalin)	1198	29	2	2	0	*	*	*		*		Suspected carcinogen.
Formamide	–	–	–	–	–							Essential for drug production.
Formic acid (Methanoic acid)	1779	60	3	2	0		*	*			*	Produces poison gas while burning; rubber overclothing required.
Hexane	1208	27	1	3	0	*	*			*		
Hydrochloric acid	1789	60	3	0	0		*	*			*	Produces poison gas while burning.
Hydrocyanic acid (Hydrogen cyanide)	1051	13	4	4	2	*	*				*	
Hydrogen, gaseous	1049	22	0	4	0	*	*				*	
Iodine	–	–	–	–	–		*	*	*			

TABLE B-1

Chemicals used in clandestine drug labs—cont'd

Chemical	UN number	ERG number	Health hazard rating	Flammability hazard rating	Reactivity hazard rating	Explosive	Poisonous	Corrosive	Precursor	Solvent	Reagent	Comments
Lead acetate	1616	53	–	–	–		*		*			Rubber overclothing required.
Lithium aluminum hydride	1410	40	3	1	2	*	*	*			*	Avoid water; rubber overclothing required.
Mercuric chloride	1624	53	–	–	–		*				*	Rubber overclothing required.
Methanamine (Methylamine)	1061	19	3	4	0	*	*	*	*	*		
Methanamine, anhydrous (Methylamine, anhydrous)	1061	19	3	4	0			*	*			Produces poison gas while burning.
Methanol (Methyl alcohol)	1230	28	1	3	0	*	*	*		*		
α-[1-(Methylamino) ethyl] benzene-methanol (Ephedrine)	–	–	–	–	–				*			Suspected carcinogen.
Methylbenzene (Toluene)	1294	27	2	3	0	*	*	*		*		Suspected carcinogen.
Morpholine (Diethylene imidoxide)	2054	29	2	3	0					*		
Nitric acid, nonfuming, concentration >40%	2031	44	3	0	0			*	*		*	Produces poison gas while burning; chemical protective suit required.
Nitroethane	2842	26	1	3	3	*	*	*	*			Produces poison gas while burning.
1,1'-Oxybisethane (Ethyl ether)	1155	26	2	4	1	*	*	*		*		
Oxybismethane (Dimethyl ether)	1039	26	2	4	1	*	*	*		*		
Phenyl-2-propanone (P2P)	–	26	1	3	0		*	*	*			Classified as a controlled substance.
Phosphoric acid	1805	60	2	0	0			*			*	

Continued.

TABLE B-1

Chemicals used in clandestine drug labs—cont'd

Chemical	UN number	ERG number	Health hazard rating	Flammability hazard rating	Reactivity hazard rating	Explosive	Poisonous	Corrosive	Precursor	Solvent	Reagent	Comments
Phosphorus pentachloride	1086	39	–	–	–		*	*			*	Avoid water.
Phosphorus trichloride	–	–	–	–	–			*			*	Avoid water.
Phosphoryl chloride (Phosphorus oxychloride)	1810	39	3	0	2		*	*			*	Avoid water.
Piperidine (Hexahydropyridine)	2401	29	–	–	–					*		
Potassium hydroxide	1813	60	3	0	1		*	*		*		
2-Propanol (Isopropyl alcohol)	1219	26	1	3	0	*	*	*		*		
2-Propanone (Acetone)	1090	26	1	3	0	*	*	*		*		
Pyridine	1282	26	2	3	0	*	*	*			*	Suspected carcinogen; chemical protective suit required.
Pyrrolidine	1922	29	–	–	–						*	Highly flammable.
Sodium	1428	40	3	1	2							Avoid water; rubber overclothing required.
Sodium acetate	–	–	–	–	–					*		
Sodium amalgam	1424	40	–	–	–	*	*	*			*	Avoid water.
Sodium bisulfate, solid	1821	60	–	–	–		*	*			*	Produces poison gas while burning.
Sodium hydroxide, dry, solid (Draino)	1823	60	3	0	1		*	*			*	Produces poison gas while burning; rubber overclothing required.
Sulfuric acid	1830	39	3	0	2		*	*			*	Reacts violently with water; rubber overclothing required.
Tetrachloromethane (Carbon tetrachloride)	1846	55	3	0	0		*	*			*	Produces poison gas while burning.

TABLE B-1

Chemicals used in clandestine drug labs—cont'd

Chemical	UN number	ERG number	Health hazard rating	Flammability hazard rating	Reactivity hazard rating	Explosive	Poisonous	Corrosive	Precursor	Solvent	Reagent	Comments
Thionyl chloride	1836	39	3	0	2		*	*			*	Reacts violently with water; rubber over-clothing required.
Thorium nitrate, solid	9171	64	1	0	0		*	*			*	Chemical is radioactive; produces poison gas while burning.
o-Toluidine	1708	55	3	2	0		*				*	
Trichloromethane (Chloroform)	1888	55	2	0	0		*	*		*		Produces poison gas while burning.
Zinc	–	–	0	1	1						*	Used as a catalyst in the reaction.

APPENDIX C

EMTAC BASIC TRAINING CURRICULUM

1. Orientation (8 hours)
   A. Role and responsibilities
   B. Policies, procedures, rules, regulations, and standard operating procedures.
      1. EMTAC
      2. Rapides Parish Sheriff's Department
      3. Tactical unit
      4. Other participating agencies
   C. Law enforcement tactical operations
      1. Why?
      2. Possible missions
      3. Organization
      4. Principles
      5. Tactics
   D. Introduction to local tactical units
      1. Rapides Parish Sheriff's Tactical Unit
      2. Louisiana State Police Tactical Unit
      3. U.S. Marshals' Service Special Operations Group and U.S. Marshals' Service Special Operations Group Training Center
      4. Louisiana State Police Criminal Investigation Bureau—North Narcotics Task Force
      5. Central Louisiana Narcotics Task Force

2. Terrorism (8 hours)
   A. Incidence of terrorist activity
   B. Possible terrorist scenarios
   C. Potential terrorist threats and targets in the area
   D. EMS and terrorism: a survival course
   E. The trauma of violence

3. Use and Care of Equipment (4 hours)
   A. Individual equipment
   B. Team equipment

4. Medical Aspects (4 hours)
   A. Team medical protocols
   B. Medical care standard operating procedures
   C. Review of principles for major trauma care

5. Support-Weapon Familiarization (8 hours classroom and range firing)
   A. Semiautomatic rifle—AR-15
   B. Police slide-action shotgun—Ithaca Model 37 (military and police)
   C. Submachine guns
      1. Heckler and Koch MP-5
      2. Ingram MAC-10

6. Handgun Marksmanship (8 hours)
   A. Principles of handgun accuracy (classroom instruction)
   B. Safety
   C. Louisiana Police Officer Survival Training (POST) handgun qualification course

7. Stress Shooting (8 hours)
   A. Lethal force—legal aspects
      1. Louisiana law
      2. Rapides Parish Sheriff's Department policy
   B. Shoot; don't shoot decisions (includes videotape simulation exercise)
   C. Handgun stress course

8. Water Survival (4 hours)
   A. 200-meter swim
   B. Floating and drown-proofing
   C. Field expedient-flotation devices

9. Tactical Movement (8 hours)
   A. Moving through obstacles
   B. Cover and concealment
   C. Arm and hand signals

10. Rappelling (8 hours)
    A. Ropes and knots
    B. Tying off to the building
    C. Basic rappelling
       1. Carabiners
       2. Figure eight
       3. Swiss or ranger seat
       4. Tactical harness
    D. Tying off and performing tasks
    E. Rappelling in full gear: includes gas mask, handgun and gun belt, load-bearing vests, and/or medic bag

11. Law Enforcement Small Unit Tactics (12 hours)
    A. Formations
    B. Ambushes and immediate action drills
    C. Scouting and patrolling

12. Hostage Negotiations (8 hours)

13. Land Navigation (6 hours)
    A. Map reading
    B. Military coordinate system
    C. Compass

14. Building Entries and Searches
    A. Classroom (4 hours)
       1. Methods
       2. Techniques
    B. Practical exercises (14 hours)
       1. Demonstrations
       2. Wax bullet and plastic target exercises: six building entry, movement, and search scenarios (with critique)
       3. Rubber bullet exercises using aggressor teams

15. Explosive Search, Safety, and Recognition (4 hours)
    A. Recognition of common explosive devices
    B. Bomb search techniques
    C. Safety precautions

16. Gases (4 hours)
    A. Agents
    B. Dispersal systems
    C. Gas mask

17. Night Handgun Shooting (4 hours)
    A. Principles
    B. Night firing course

18. Helicopter Operations (4 hours)
   A. Landing zone preparation
   B. Loading and unloading
   C. Insertion and extraction (includes patient evacuation)
   D. Safety

19. Officer Down (4 hours)
   A. Scenarios
   B. Immediate action drill

20. Practical Scenario (8 hours)
   Run with a law enforcement agency tactical unit; includes tactical movement to the objective, building entry in which a team member is critically injured, building search to locate the member, immediate stabilization and removal, and more definitive stabilization and evacuation (videotaped for critique).

This training outline is used by Rapides Parish, Alexandria, Louisiana, to instruct SWAT medics. *(Courtesy Stephen K. Erwin, EMTAC Team Leader, Rapides Parish Sheriff's Department, Alexandria, La.)*

▼   ▼

APPENDIX D

EMTAC EQUIPMENT

Figures D-1, D-2, D-3, and the box show items of personal equipment, team equipment, and medical supplies issued to members of the Rapides Parish, Louisiana, EMTAC team. Although this equipment presently meets the needs of an EMTAC team, it is not inclusive of all the equipment needed for every situation. The items in the box are an example of the type and quantity of equipment that supports SWAT operations. Do not carry or use any items listed in the box that are not approved by your department head or medical director.

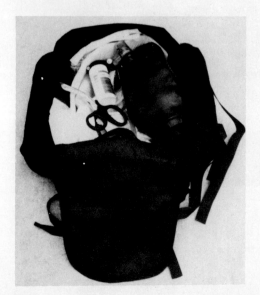

FIGURE D-1
EMTAC individual medical bag.
(Courtesy Rapides Parish Sheriff's Department, Alexandria, La.)

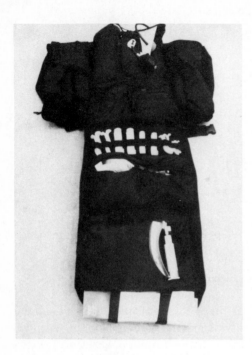

FIGURE D-2
EMTAC team medical bag. *(Courtesy Rapides Parish Sheriff's Department, Alexandria, La.)*

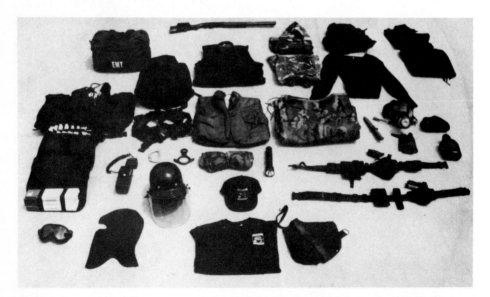

FIGURE D-3
Equipment carried by SWAT medics of the Rapides Parish Sheriff's Department.
(Courtesy Rapides Parish Sheriff's Department, Alexandria, La.)

EMTAC EQUIPMENT

UNIFORMS
Black military-type, two-piece battle dress utility uniform (BDU)
Black nylon web belt with subdued buckle
Black crew-neck t-shirt
Black nylon knit or mesh baseball-style cap
Black combat (tactical response) boots
Heavy-duty boot socks (at least two pairs)
Black military-type field jacket with liner
Black and orange MA-1 bomber jacket (optional)
Black "woolly-pully" sweater
Black "Navy" watch cap
Camouflage poncho with liner
Gloves (insulated or wool)
Undergarments and socks (depending on weather conditions)

ARMAMENT

Handguns

Colt or Smith and Wesson .357 Magnum, double-action revolver with 3- or 4-inch barrel
Smith and Wesson 9 mm × 19 mm NATO double-action, semiautomatic pistol

Reloading devices

Revolver: A minimum of 4 speed loaders
Semiautomatic pistol: A minimum of 2 magazines

Ammunition

Use Winchester Silvertip, Remington Peters, Federal, or CCI Lawman cartridges.
Revolver: 110 or 125 grain, jacketed hollow-point +P cartridges
Semiautomatic pistol: 110 grain, jacketed hollow-point +P cartridges

Belt, holsters, and carriers

Black, ballistic, nylon pistol belt with snap buckle
Black, ballistic, nylon pancake holster for handgun
Revolver: Two black, ballistic, nylon, dual-speed loader carriers
Semiautomatic pistol: Black, ballistic, nylon magazine carrier

PERSONAL EQUIPMENT
Kershaw "Black Horse" folding lock-blade survival knife in black, nylon carrier
Two D-cell-capacity Mag-lites or flashlight with four alkaline batteries and two krypton
  bulbs
Symplex black, nylon tactical rappelling harness
Black, anodized steel carabiner
Black Assault 8 descender
Black, leather rappelling gloves
Two gear bags (equipment bags)
Black, nylon, mesh load-bearing vest
ALS trauma kit in black, nylon rucksack
Gas mask with filters and carrying case
Soft body armor
Pager
Watch
Sunglasses
Two 1-quart military canteens with black covers
Assault rescue belt
Large, tactical rappelling gear pouch

Continued.

APPENDIX D

EMTAC EQUIPMENT — CONT'D

TEAM EQUIPMENT

Equipment	Quantity
ALS trauma kit packed in a Brigade-Quartermaster Emergency Med-bag 84	1
ALS trauma kit packed in a Group 5 Para-rescue Pack A	1
VHF high-band, hand-held radio transceivers (5-watt, 4-channel—both EMS and law enforcement) with flexible, rubber antennas, lapel microphone, earplug, extra battery and charger, and tactical case	3
150-foot by ½-inch black, kermantle rappelling ropes in tactical rope bags	2
300-foot by ½-inch black, kermantle rappelling rope in tactical rope bag	1
Folding scoop stretcher with black, nylon straps	1
Olive-drab (OD) blanket	1
Case of 1000 ml bags of Ringer's lactate*	1
Blood administration sets*	12
Bag of 36 intravenous catheters (large-bore angiocaths or similar)*	1

ALS TRAUMA KIT (INDIVIDUAL AND TEAM)

Equipment	Quantity
IV set-ups: 1000 ml bag of Ringer's lactate with blood administration set, 14-gauge, 16-gauge, and 18-gauge intravenous catheters (one of each), 2 alcohol preps, and 2 Betadine preps; secured to the IV bag with a rubber tourniquet	2
8- by 10-inch ABD pads	6
4- by 4-inch gauze sponges	12
Rolls of 6-ply, 4½-inch by 4¹⁄₁₀-yard Kerlix bandage	6
Rolls of 3-inch by 5-yard Kling bandage	6
Roll of 3-inch by 10-yard adhesive tape	1
Rolls of 1-inch by 10-yard cloth hypoallergenic tape	2
3- by 18-inch petroleum gauze patch dressings	6
Stethoscope	1
Blood pressure cuff	1
Endotracheal intubation kit: laryngoscope with straight blade and curved blade, two 7.5 mm endotracheal tubes, stylet, 10 ml syringe, roll of 1-inch tape, and Endolock (or similar paramedic tube restraint)	1
Esophageal obturator airway kit: mask, airway tube, foil envelopes of K-Y lubricant, and 35 ml syringe	1
Large EMT shears	1
½-inch Lister bandage scissors	5

*Items stored together in a foot locker and placed in any available vehicle for transport.

EMTAC EQUIPMENT—CONT'D

ALS TRAUMA KIT (INDIVIDUAL AND TEAM)—CONT'D

Equipment	Quantity
Triangular bandages (2 safety pins each)	6
1- by 3-inch Band-Aids	25
Alcohol preps	12
Betadine preps	12
10 ml syringes	2
3 ml syringes	4
18-gauge by 1½-inch hypodermic needles	2
21-gauge by 1½-inch hypodermic needles	2
23-gauge by 1-inch hypodermic needles	2
Bermann 100 mm oral pharyngeal airways	2
Bermann 90 mm oral pharyngeal airways	2
Bermann 80 mm oral pharyngeal airways	2
Bermann 60 mm oral pharyngeal airways	2
Bermann 40 mm oral pharyngeal airways	2
Hudson lifesaver kit	1
Pocket mask	1
Bite sticks	2
Ammonia inhalants	12
Mini-mag penlight with spare batteries and spare bulb	1
Tubex syringe	1

ALS EQUIPMENT IN TEAM TRAUMA KIT

Pharmacopeia	Quantity
Sodium bicarbonate ampules, mEq (Bristoljet or equal)	2
1:1000 Adrenalin ampules	2
1:10000 Epinephrine ampules (Bristoljet or equal)	2
0.1 mg/ml 10 ml Atropine ampules (Bristoljet or equal)	2

ALS EQUIPMENT IN GROUP 5 PARA-RESCUE PACK A

Equipment	Quantity
MAST kit with foot pump	1
Disposable bag-valve mask ventilation unit	1
50 mg Dramamine ampules	5
¼-grain morphine sulfate ampules (drawn from pharmacy at time of mission)	5

NOTES

Preface

[1] In 1980 Michael A. Olds had been a paramedic for the Baltimore City Fire Department for 6 months. His partner on Medic 16 (a seasoned firefighter) had stressed the need to avoid standing in front of a door of a residence when knocking. During a response to an injured person in a row house in west Baltimore, the two paramedics were knocking on the door of a residence when two arrows were shot through the closed door. Because they were standing to the side of the door, neither firefighter was injured. They backed away from the residence, and the police department secured the scene. Olds MA: Interview by Krebs DR, Baltimore, 20 June 1988.

[2] National Fire Academy: 1988 US firefighter fatalities, Emmitsburg, Md, 1988, photocopy.

[3] New Orleans Department of Police: What happened. . ., Our Beat 24(1):3, 1973.

[4] Weslager J: Paramedic assault, Emergency, The Journal of Emergency Services 15(15):13, 1983.

[5] San Diego Fire Department: McDonald's restaurant critique, 2 Oct 1984, photocopy.

[6] Scott F: Caught in the crossfire, Advance for Respiratory Therapists Jan 1989, newsletter.

Chapter 1

[1] News and Trends, Fire Chief 33(3):12, 1989.

[2] American Body Armor & Equipment, Inc: Second generation, light-weight body armor, Emergency Medical Services 16(3):61, 1987, advertisement.

[3] Protection Development International Corp: Antiterrorist cab, Fire Chief 32(8):66, 1988, advertisement.

Chapter 2

[1]Cab forward apparatus do not protect personnel in the front seat with the engine block, but no matter what type of cab you are using, follow the same positioning procedures.

[2]Maryland State Police Street Survival School, State Police Training Academy: Pikesville, Md, Aug 1983, classroom notes.

Chapter 3

[1]Ludington G: Interview by Gabriele M, Baltimore, Md, 18 Sept 1988.

[2]Beard RJ: Stop made in June 1981, Interview by Gabriele M, 21 March 1989.

[3]Ennis Sr WS: Fire and EMS personnel from the West Carrollton Fire Department on the scene, Interview by Henry KC, 19 March 1989.

[4]Description of a vehicle with steel-plating, gun ports, bullet-proof glass and tires, tear-gas launchers, and an oil tank that dumps oil on the roadway when activated. Arizona Department of Public Safety: Criminal intelligence information bulletin Pub No 88-07, 22 July 1988.

Chapter 4

[1]US Department of Justice, Federal Bureau of Investigation: Uniform crime reports, 1986, Federal Bureau of Investigation Pub No 181-487:60532, Washington, DC, 1987, US Government Printing Office.

[2]Lovette E: Carrying duty ammo for revolvers, New Mexico Lawman Jan 1977, photocopy; and in Adams RJ, McTernan TM, and Remsberg C: Street survival, Northbrook, Ill, 1987, Calibre Press.

[3]Maryland State Police In-Service Training School for Trooper First Class: 1983.

[4]Maryland State Police troopers wear Stetson uniform hats that are similar to those worn by military drill instructors.

[5]Maryland State Police In-Service Training School for Officer Survival: 1987.

Chapter 5

[1]Fire Specialist Bruce A. Snyder, Baltimore County Fire Department, is a former member of the Baltimore City Fire Department where he was assigned to Truck 12. On the night of 8 September 1982, he was detailed to Engine 46. He was one of the firefighters on the scene of this incident. Snyder BA: Interview by Krebs DR, 16 July 1988.

Chapter 6

[1]On 20 April 1987, ambulance personnel from the Elkridge Volunteer Fire Department, Maryland, knocked on the door of a mobile home in the Capitol Mobile Home Park. Without warning, the occupant of the mobile home fired an arrow through the closed door, barely missing the ambulance crew. Kiesling P: Interview by Krebs DR, 13 Apr 1988.

[2]Some volunteers on the eastern shore of Maryland live so far from the fire station or squad quarters that they report directly to the scene of the emergency in their personal vehicles. In one situation, a firefighter was the first person to arrive on the scene of a rescue call in a rural residence. He rushed through the open front door to find an elderly couple sitting in their front room with looks of surprise and fear. "Did you call the fire department?" he

asked. "No," they replied. He was in the wrong house. Student: Interview by Krebs DR, Oct 1983.

[3] While Dennis Krebs was responding to calls in a medic unit with the Baltimore City Fire Department, he often experienced occupants shutting and blocking doors behind the rescue team after they entered a room to treat the patient. At times the rescue team had to fight their way out of the room physically. The medical-assist call discussed in Chapter 5 by Fire Specialist Bruce A. Snyder was a setup to lure fire and police personnel into an ambush.

[4] Gabriele and Krebs were involved in this incident when they responded as paramedics with the Rosedale Volunteer Fire Company, Baltimore County, Maryland.

[5] Incledon PJ: Know the risk: window entry, With New York Firefighters 49(2):22, 1988.

Chapter 7

[1] Fite R and Sauer E: 1 dead, 2 injured, The Sentinel, p 1, 30 May 1987.

[2] Fite R and Strong K: Second victim of shooting dies, The Sentinel, p 1, 3 June 1987.

Chapter 8

[1] Actual experience of Dennis R. Krebs.

[2] Adams RJ, McTernan TM, and Remsberg C: Street survival, Northbrook, Ill, 1987, Calibre Press.

Chapter 9

[1] San Diego Fire Department: McDonald's restaurant critique, 2 Oct 1984.

[2] Burke TW: Officer survival: the ricocheting bullet, unpublished term paper, Washington, DC, 18 Apr 1984, photocopy.

Chapter 10

[1] Vayer JS and Plitt KW: Siege, Firehouse, 7:71, Sept 1982.

[2] Remsberg C: The tactical edge, Northbrook, Ill, 1987, Calibre Press.

[3] Hogewood W: Hostage taking, Beltsville, Md, 1988, Prince Georges County Police Department, Special Operations Division, photocopy.

[4] Kobetz RW and Cooper HA: Target terrorism. Paper presented to the meeting of the International Association of Chiefs of Police, Gaithersburg, Md, 1978, International Association of Chiefs of Police.

[5] Hogewood, p 2.

[6] Fuselier GW: A practical overview of hostage negotiations, FBI Law Enforcement Bulletin 50:2, June/July 1981.

[7] Fuselier, p 2.

[8] Hildreth R: Terrorism, Law and Order Magazine 36(6):41, 1988.

[9] Strentz T: A hostage psychological survival guide, FBI Law Enforcement Bulletin 47(11):1, 1978.

[10] Kobetz, p 80.

[11] Strentz, p 3.

[12] Bolz Jr FA: How to be a hostage and live, Secaucus, NJ, 1987, Lyle Stuart, Inc.

[13] Bolz, p 13.

[14] Lang D: A reporter at large, New Yorker, p 56, Nov 1974.

[15]Strentz T: Law enforcement policy and ego defense of the hostage, FBI Law Enforcement Bulletin, 48(4):7, 1979.

[16]Fuselier, p 6.

Chapter 11

[1]Lenz RR: Explosives and bomb disposal guide, Springfield, Ill, 1971, Charles C Thomas.

[2]US Department of the Treasury, Bureau of Alcohol, Tobacco, and Firearms: Explosive incidents report, 1986, Bureau of Alcohol, Tobacco, and Firearms Pub No 5400, Washington, DC, 1987, US Government Printing Office.

[3]Lenz, p 15.

[4]Stoffel J: Explosives and homemade bombs, ed 2, Springfield, Ill, 1972, Charles C Thomas.

[5]Lenz, p 16.

[6]Stoffel, p 36.

[7]Prince Georges County Fire Department, Prince Georges County, Md: Standard operating procedure 3.00.

[8]Stoffel, p 117.

[9]Ennis Sr WS: Interview by Henry KC, 6 Jan 1989.

Chapter 12

[1]New York Times News Service: DEA issues warning as more makeshift labs turn out methamphetamine, Baltimore Sun, p 6, 4 Dec 1988.

[2]Beaty J: Tales of the crank trade, Time, p 10, 24 Apr 1989.

[3]New York Times News Service, p 6.

[4]Siel R: 1986 Oregon laboratory seizures, report, Feb 1988, Western States Information Network.

[5]Molino Sr LN: Clandestine drug labs-Part I, what's brewing, The Pennsylvania Fireman 52(5):60, Jan 1989.

[6]Frye M: Clandestine drug labs and the first responder, Speaking of Fire Winter:2, 1988.

[7]Sacramento Fire Department: Clandestine drug lab incidents: procedures for HMRT, Sacramento, Calif, 1 Feb 1987, photocopy.

Chapter 14

[1]Neale R: SWAT team paramedics, JEMS 5(2):39, 1980.

[2]City of Miami Department of Fire and Rescue: Standard operating procedures: SWAT medic program, Miami, photocopy.

[3]Rapides Parish Sheriff's Department: EMTAC rules and regulations, Rapides Parish, La, photocopy.

[4]Essex MJ: Personal communication to Erwin SK, 19 Dec 1985.

[5]City of Miami Department of Fire and Rescue, p 3.

Appendix A

[1]Weslager J: Paramedic assault, Emergency, The Journal of Emergency Services 15(15):13, 1983.

[2]Bamatree WR: Letter to Reincke PH, Towson, Md, 27 Oct 1988.

[3]Safariland Ballistics Industries: Gall's holiday gift catalog C3:30, 1988, advertisement.

[4]A 40-page catalog devoted to "the world's best SWAT and hostage rescue team clothing and equipment," now includes emergency medical bags and a med-bag accessory pouch. Tactical action gear, Brigade Quartermaster, Tactical Catalog 17, 1988/1989.

[5]Miner LH: Ballistic testing of used soft body armor of Kevlar aramid, Wilmington, Del, 1987, EI Du Pont De Nemours & Co, Industrial Fibers Division, photocopy.

[6]EI Du Pont De Nemours & Co, Industrial Fibers Division, Textile Fibers Department: Dress for survival, Kevlar personal body armor facts book, ed 3, Wilmington, Del, 1987, EI Du Pont De Nemours & Co.

[7]FBI statistics indicate that the percentage of police officers killed with .357 Magnum and 9 mm handguns rose from 13% in 1974 to 35% in 1984. EI Du Pont de Nemours & Co, Industrial Fibers Division, Textile Fibers Department: Dress for survival, Kevlar personal body armor facts book, ed 3, Wilmington, Del, 1987, EI Du Pont De Nemours & Co.

[8]EI Du Pont De Nemours & Co, p 3.

BIBLIOGRAPHY

Adams RJ, McTernan TM, and Remsberg C: Street survival, Northbrook, Ill, 1987, Calibre Press.

American Body Armor & Equipment, Inc: Second generation, light-weight body armor, Emergency Medical Services 16(3):61, 1987, advertisement.

Arizona Department of Public Safety: Criminal intelligence information bulletin Pub No 88-07, 22 July 1988.

Bamatree WR: Letter to Reincke PH, Towson, Md, 27 Oct 1988.

Beard RJ: Interview by Gabriele M, 21 March 1989.

Beaty J: Tales of the crank trade, Time, p 10, 24 Apr 1989.

Bolz Jr FA: How to be a hostage and live, Secaucus, NJ, 1987, Lyle Stuart, Inc.

Burke TW: Officer survival: the ricocheting bullet, unpublished term paper, Washington, DC, 18 Apr 1984, photocopy.

EI Du Pont De Nemours & Co, Industrial Fibers Division, Textile Fibers Department: Dress for survival, Kevlar personal body armor facts book, ed 3, Wilmington, Del, 1987, EI Du Pont De Nemours & Co.

Ennis Sr WS: Interview by Henry KC, 6 Jan 1989.

Ennis Sr WS: Interview by Henry KC, 19 March 1989.

Essex MJ: Letter to Krebs DR, Abingdon, Md, 19 Dec 1985.

Fite R and Sauer E: 1 dead, 2 injured, The Sentinel, p 1, 30 May 1987.

Fite R and Strong K: Second victim of shooting dies, The Sentinel, p 1, 3 June 1987.

Frye M: Clandestine drug labs and the first responder, Speaking of Fire Winter:2, 1988.

Fuselier GW: A practical overview of hostage negotiations, FBI Law Enforcement Bulletin 50:2, June/July 1981.

Hildreth R: Terrorism, Law and Order Magazine 36(6):41, 1988.

Hogewood W: Hostage taking, Beltsville, Md, 1988, Prince Georges County Police Department, Special Operations Division, photocopy.

Incledon PJ: Know the risk: window entry, With New York Firefighters 49(2):22, 1988.

Kobetz RW and Cooper HA: Target terrorism. Paper presented to the International Association of Chiefs of Police, Gaithersburg, Md, 1978, International Association of Chiefs of Police.

Lang D: A reporter at large, New Yorker, p 56, Nov 1974.

Lenz RR: Explosives and bomb disposal guide, Springfield, Ill, 1971, Charles C Thomas.

Miami Fire Department: Standard operating procedures: SWAT medic program, Miami, photocopy.

Miner LH: Ballistic testing of used soft body armor of Kevlar aramid, Wilmington, Del, 1987, EI Du Pont De Nemours & Co, Industrial Fibers Division, photocopy.

Molino Sr LN: Clandestine drug labs-Part I, what's brewing, The Pennsylvania Fireman 52(5):60, 1989.

National Fire Protection Association: Fire protection guide on hazardous materials, ed 9, Quincy, Mass, 1986, National Fire Protection Association.

Neale R: SWAT team paramedics, JEMS 5(2):39, 1980.

New Orleans Department of Police: What happened. . ., Our Beat 24(1):3, 1973.

News and Trends, Fire Chief 33(3):12, 1989.

New York Times News Service: DEA issues warning as more makeshift labs turn out methamphetamine, Baltimore Sun, p 6, 4 Dec 1988.

Olds MA: Interview by Krebs DR, Baltimore, 20 June 1988.

Protection Development International Corp: Antiterrorist cab, Fire Chief 32(8):66, 1988, advertisement.

Rapides Parish Sheriff's Department: EMTAC rules and regulations, Rapides Parish, La, photocopy.

Remsberg C: The tactical edge, Northbrook, Ill, 1987, Calibre Press.

Sacramento Fire Department: Clandestine drug lab incidents: procedures for HMRT, Sacramento, Calif, 1 Feb 1987, photocopy.

Safariland Ballistics Industries: Gall's holiday gift catalog C3:30, 1988, advertisement.

San Diego Fire Department: McDonald's restaurant critique, 2 Oct 1984, photocopy.

Scott F: Caught in the crossfire, Advance for Respiratory Therapists Jan 1989, newsletter.

Siel R: 1986 Oregon laboratory seizures report, Feb 1988, Western States Information Network.

Snyder BA: Interview by Krebs DR, 16 July 1988.

Stoffel J: Explosives and homemade bombs, ed 2, Springfield, Ill, 1972, Charles C Thomas.

Strentz T: A hostage psychological survival guide, FBI Law Enforcement Bulletin 47(11):1, 1978.

Strentz T: Law enforcement policy and ego defense of the hostage, FBI Law Enforcement Bulletin 48(4):7, 1979.

Tactical action gear, Brigade Quartermaster, Tactical Catalog 17, 1988/1989.

US Department of Justice, Federal Bureau of Investigation: Uniform crime reports, 1986, Federal Bureau of Investigation Pub No 181-487:60532, Washington, DC, 1987, US Government Printing Office.

US Department of Transportation, Office of Hazardous Materials Transportation: Emergency response guidebook, Department of Transportation Pub No 5800, Washington, DC, 1987, US Government Printing Office.

US Department of the Treasury, Bureau of Alcohol, Tobacco, and Firearms: Bomb and physical security planning, Bureau of Alcohol, Tobacco, and Firearms Pub No 7550, Washington, DC, 1987, US Government Printing Office.

US Department of the Treasury, Bureau of Alcohol, Tobacco, and Firearms: Explosive incidents report, 1986, Bureau of Alcohol, Tobacco, and Firearms Pub No 5400, Washington, DC, 1987, US Government Printing Office.

Vayer JS and Plitt KW: Siege, Firehouse 7:71, Sept 1982.

Weslager J: Paramedic assault, Emergency, The Journal of Emergency Services 15(15):13, 1983.

▼   ▼

ABOUT THE AUTHORS

Dennis R. Krebs joined the fire service as a volunteer with the Pikesville Volunteer Fire Company, Baltimore County, Maryland, in 1974. The same year he began working for the Baltimore City Fire Department as a firefighter. In 1979 he joined the Baltimore County Fire Department, where he is currently a lieutenant in the Fire Suppression Division.

Dennis is a codeveloper of the highly successful Medical Emergency Defense and Incident Control (MEDIC) Seminar on which this book is based. He has presented this seminar to fire, rescue, and emergency medical service organizations throughout the United States since 1983. He serves as an adjunct faculty member with the Baltimore County Fire Department.

Dennis is certified in accordance with the National Fire Protection Association's Standards as Fire Officer IV and Instructor III. He is a member of the International Society of Fire Service Instructors and, as a member of the American Society for Testing and Materials, serves on the Coordinating Committee on Flash Point and Related Properties.

Kenneth C. Henry began his fire service career as a volunteer in Baltimore County in 1955. In 1973 he was fire chief of the Brandon Fire Department, Brandon, Florida. In 1979 the Brandon Fire Department merged with the Hillsborough County Fire Department, and Chief Henry became district chief in the Suppression Division. He is a life member of the Woodlawn Volunteer Fire Company in Baltimore County and The Fellowship of Christian Firefighters International.

Chief Henry's education includes an associate in science in fire administration (honors) from St. Petersburg Junior College and a bachelor of arts in political science and master of public administration degrees from the University of South Florida. He is a member of the National Political Science Honor Society (Pi Sigma Alpha), the Golden Key National Honor Society, and the American Society for Public Administration.

As an active member of the International Society of Fire Service Instructors, Ken has served on task forces studying problems facing the fire service. He specializes in project management for program development, technical research and writing, and fire department analysis.

Mark B. Gabriele is an 11-year veteran of the Maryland State Police. He is currently assigned as a sergeant in the Aviation Division as the training coordinator for the medical staff. He is responsible for entrance level and continuing education for flight paramedics assigned to the division.

Mark began his career assigned to the Field Operations Bureau performing complete law-enforcement services. He transferred to the Aviation Division and served as a flight paramedic before moving to the training section.

Mark has been an active volunteer firefighter with the Rosedale Volunteer Fire Company in Baltimore County since 1975. He is certified in accordance with the National Fire Protection Association's Standards as Fire Fighter II. He is listed on the national registry as an Emergency Medical Technician-Paramedic and is a certified Maryland Paramedic Instructor.

Mark is a codeveloper of the highly successful Medical Emergency Defense and Incident Control (MEDIC) Seminar on which this book is based. He has presented this seminar to fire, rescue, and emergency medical service organizations throughout the United States since 1983. He is an active member of the National Flight Paramedics Association, the Association of Air Medical Services, and the Maryland Critical Incident–Stress Debriefing Team.

INDEX